WHY NATURAL THERAPIES WORK

AND HOW TO MAKE THEM WORK BETTER

The UNI-SYN Method

C. P. NEGRI, OMD, ND

Why Natural Therapies Work and How To Make Them Work Better The Uni-Syn Method

By C.P. Negri, OMD, ND
First Edition

Printed in the United States of America.

ISBN: 978-1-7372929-3-7

also by C. P. NEGRI:

Green Medicine
Naturopathic Treatment of Blood Pressure
Naturopathic Treatment of Emotional Illness
The Negri Manual of Natural Medicine, Vol. I and Vol.II

DEDICATION

To Harry Miller, DO,
who restored my vision
and changed a detective
into a doctor

CONTENTS

FOREWORD

If you are a practitioner of medicine, whether conventional or alternative, I highly recommend reading this book.

Dr. Negri's extensive experience of over 44 years in practice, along with his exposure to a wide variety of therapies, has led him to identify commonalities among all the different areas of expertise he encountered. His concept of Uni-Syn, a unified synthesis of the elements and principles of natural laws that govern the effective application of treatments often ignored in mainstream medicine, is a testament to the wisdom and inspiration of his predecessors.

This book is a valuable addition to any practitioner's desk reference library. By absorbing the information in this book, practitioners can become more effective in their practice and gain considerable insight into the fascinating phenomena that govern the practice of medicine.

Brandon Drabek, ND

PREFACE

This book came to pass because it came to my attention repeatedly over the past forty-seven years in practice that there are laws of nature that are established and codified in the sciences—agriculture, chemistry, electricity, physics, and even animal-husbandry—laws that are relatively ignored in mainstream medicine, which ironically considers itself "science-based". On the other hand, the so-called "alternative" medical fields have all been built around many of these principles, which puts them on a scientific footing that is often unrecognized.

Medicine, both alternative and conventional, is full of made-up words that have been adopted into the language and no longer seem odd. It is with some embarrassment that I ask the world to accept one more.

Uni-Syn is a ***uni***fied ***syn***thesis of the elements involved in the effective application of such varied therapies as massage, joint manipulation, acupuncture, electrotherapy, hydrotherapy, and even the prescribing of oral medications. All consistently effective practitioners seem to be unconsciously taking advantage of natural laws that are simpler and actually more profound than the mountains of knowledge that any of these health care providers were required to digest in school. In fact, if truth be told, the best methods are usually the ones gleaned from an older and more experienced practitioner, rather than from the textbooks.

I would like to say that I was lucky in my being able to work and learn at the elbow of such veteran doctors; but the fact is, luck had nothing to do with it. I sought out older practitioners both because I had an affinity with their generation and because I felt that there was a lot of missing information when I was in school. I simply did not always get the results I expected when I applied what I had learned in school. Yet, there were some who did. I was extremely hungry for what they knew.

The true luck actually came in becoming a classical naturopath, because my exposure to our wide variety of therapies led me to gradually spot some commonalities among all the different areas of expertise that these men and women had. If I had been solely trained in manual medicine, or acupuncture, or botanical medicine, I would not have been able to perceive the essential elements common to all the experts' protocols.

Five principles guide this work: The "Three Ps" (Provocation, Polarity, and Periodicity), and two other complementary concepts. They are individually detailed later in the book; please don't cheat yourself by skipping to the back. By reading the overview of all the different therapies using these principles, one gains considerable insight.

It is my hope that whether your name is followed by ND, MD, LMT, DOM, DN, DC, DO—whatever—you will be a more effective practitioner by absorbing the information herein.

I find these phenomena intensely fascinating. I think you will, too.

C.P. Negri, OMD, ND

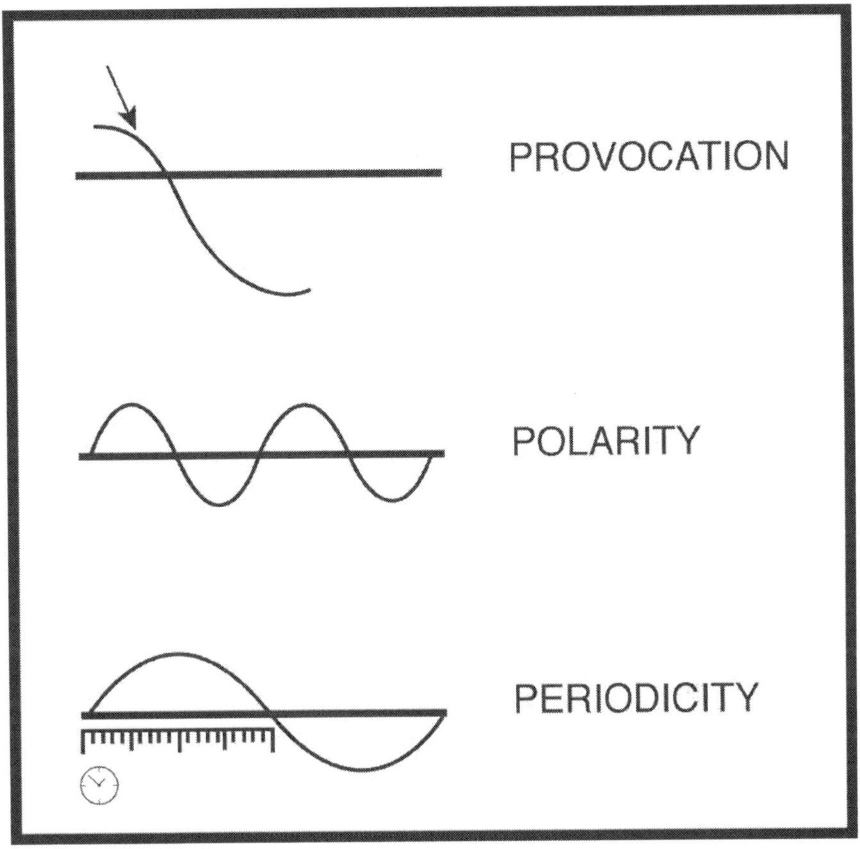
PROVOCATION
POLARITY
PERIODICITY

1

THE MYSTERIES OF ELECTRICITY

We will begin our study with an overview of the properties of electricity. This is not for the benefit of those using the various types of electro-therapy in their practices, however; it is essential to understand the physics of electricity in order to understand Uni-Syn. The reader should not pass over this chapter because it contains information that illustrates how the physical world confirms the principles expounded in this book.

The two broad categories of electric current used for therapeutic purposes are *Galvanic* and *bipolar.* They have different properties and uses, and these properties have ramifications for other types of therapy not involving electricity, including massage, acupuncture, Chiropractic, etc.

Galvanic current, named after Prof. Galvani who performed the famous experiments with frog legs, is nothing more than direct current (DC). It is the type of electricity contained in a common battery, and its use in health care derives from its polarity effects. It is a unidirectional current; that is, the two leads from the current source produce a flow of electrons in opposite directions. When this current enters the body, it breaks up some of the molecules it encounters into their component atoms (ions). All ions have a positive or negative electric charge native to them. They attract or repel other ions, depending on the polarity. Like charges repel, unlike charges attract. Neutral molecules in the body, when in contact with Galvanic current, release the positive and negative ions that formed them. Galvanic current, therefore, is capable of chemical actions.

It should be borne in mind that it is a universal law that like poles repel and unlike poles attract. And of course, without both poles present, the circuit is not completed and no electricity flows at all.

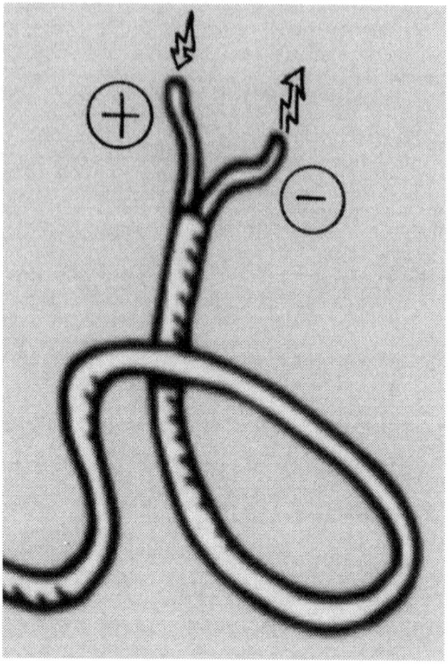

Galvanic electricity is often used medically to regenerate muscles that have become weakened through disease or injury. It can contract the muscle to which it is applied, and usually the negative pole is placed there because the negative polarity is stimulating. Conversely, the positive pole is inhibiting, and is therefore used to relax a muscle. The active pole is chosen according to the need (and the contact electrode used is always smaller then the other).

Notice that in the illustration electrons are being "pulled" by one wire in the cable and "pushed" by the other.

Actions of Galvanic Electricity

POSITIVE POLE	NEGATIVE POLE
• Sedative • Decreases congestion • Relieves pain in acute conditions • Attracts acids • Repels alkali • Contracts • Stops hemorrhage • Hardens tissues • Produces oxygen	• Stimulative • Increases congestion • Relieve pain in chronic conditions • Attracts alkali • Repels acids • Dilates • Increases blood flow • Softens tissues • Produces hydrogen

Galvanic electricity, because of its unidirectional nature and specific ion flow, can be used to introduce medicinal substances into the body without resorting to injection. This is possible because the ions of the medicinal substance are repelled by a current of the same polarity, and the resulting effect is called *iontophoresis*. Also called "ionic medication", this ion transfer is possible because of the unidirectional nature of Galvanic or DC current, and is not possible with other types of current. The advantages of this for the practitioner whose scope of practice does not include injection are obvious.

Like poles repel and unlike poles attract.

The chemical effects of electrical stimulation were proven by the classic experiment made by LeDuc where he placed two rabbits in series in a circuit of Galvanic electricity. One had an electrode soaked with strychnine sulfate attached to it, and the other rabbit had one soaked with potassium cyanide—both poisonous solutions. The electrodes between the rabbits were soaked with water. When a current was passed through the circuit with the polarity negative on the left and the polarity positive on the

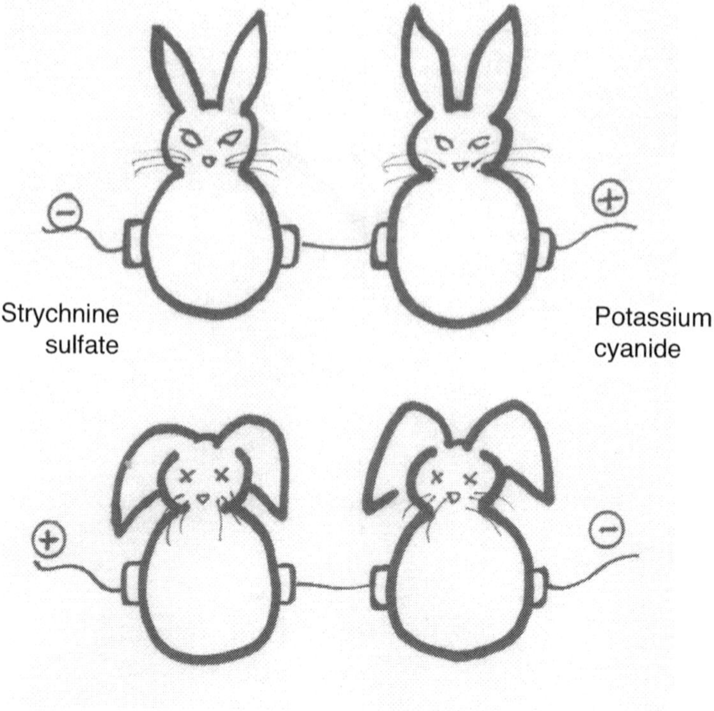

right, the rabbits were unharmed. When the polarity was reversed, both animals died quickly. This is because strychnine's ions are positively charged and cyanide's are negatively charged. It was not until the same polarity current reached each electrode with a toxic solution that the current repelled the ions and they entered the rabbits. The positive pole drove the strychnine into the one animal, and the negative pole drove the cyanide into the other.

Sinusoidal Electricity

In bipolar current, the polarity of the electricity reverses constantly, at whatever rate the generator is set. How often this occurs is the frequency. The alternating current (AC) that we all draw from for our electrical appliances is a bipolar current. In the United States, the frequency is 60 Hz. This means the polarity of each pole changes sixty times a second.

Bipolar current can be shaped into many wave forms; that is, the shape that the oscillations make if they are visualized. A square wave makes more or less a square shape on an oscilloscope. A sawtooth wave makes jagged tracings like a saw blade. These different wave forms have different characteristics. What concerns us is the wave form known as Sinusoidal current. It is named because of its shape being similar to the mathematical form, the *sine wave.* Consequently, it is typically referred to as sine wave treatment when used medically.

The sinusoidal current rhythmically rises to a peak from the zero point, then falls back to the zero point, representing a positive cycle. At that point it begins a fall into the negative cycle, where it reaches an equal maximum of a negative charge, then rises back toward the median/zero point and completes the cycle. Thus, each positive wave is followed by a negative wave. Because any chemical action of the positive wave is counteracted by the negative and vice-versa, the sinusoidal current has no net chemical effects. It is typically used to create rhythmic contractions in the muscles and also in the viscera. Most electrotherapy devices in use today in conventional medicine and physical therapy are sine wave producers (most famously the "TENS unit"). Sometimes the amplitude of the current is made to rise and fall throughout the treatment, creating another therapeutic factor. This is traditionally referred to as a *surging sine wave* treatment[1].

Sinusoidal current can have stimulating and inhibiting effects in spite of there being no fixed polarity of the electrodes. A small amount will stimulate action in the body. When the treatment is continued, it begins to inhibit action more and more from the over-stimulation, resulting in a sedating effect[2].

---

[1] Today this is referred to as a "ramped bipolar current".

[2] This is why TENS units are placed on the patient for extended use on and off throughout the day in treating chronic pain.

In this way, any stimulus that possesses no polarity in itself can be made to have differing effects by the force with which it is applied and for the length of time applied. For example, in Hydrotherapy, a stimulating effect is gained from either hot or cold water—if applied for a short length of time. One would think that hot and cold would have opposite effects, and they do; however, their length of application results in a common effect. A long hot, or cold, application of water is generally depressive and will inhibit many processes while a short application stimulates[3]. This also goes for manual therapies, acupuncture, and even the administration of medicines, as we shall see later.

Piezoelectricity

Piezoelectricity is electricity resulting from pressure, *piezo* being derived from the Greek word for pressure. It is the interaction between the mechanical and electrical properties of certain materials, most notably quartz crystals, but also 22 other organic materials. The crystal is struck sharply and rapidly with a plunger within a cylinder, causing the walls of the crystal to waver, and the resulting brief voltage emits a spark of electric current from an opening, like a spark plug in an automobile.

As for the other organic materials that act similarly: Wood, silk, and enamel can generate a small electric charge when mechanically stressed, but also (and more pertinent for our purposes) *tissues within the human body likewise produce piezoelectricity.* Bone, the dentin in teeth, tendons, fascia, and collagen have been found to have piezoelectric capacity.

Piezoelectric devices commonly used are in fireplace igniters, cigarette lighters, inkjet printers, loudspeakers, and atomic force microscopes. But there are lesser-known devices for using piezoelectricity for health purposes. Implements to apply a charge of current to acupuncture points have been

---

[3] Boyle and Saine, *Principles of Hydrotherapy*, p.48

around for some time, although they are not typically used in the acupuncture profession.

This will be expanded upon in later chapters, but the basics of this phenomenon belonged in this chapter along with other types of electricity.

2

THE MANIPULATIVE PROFESSIONS

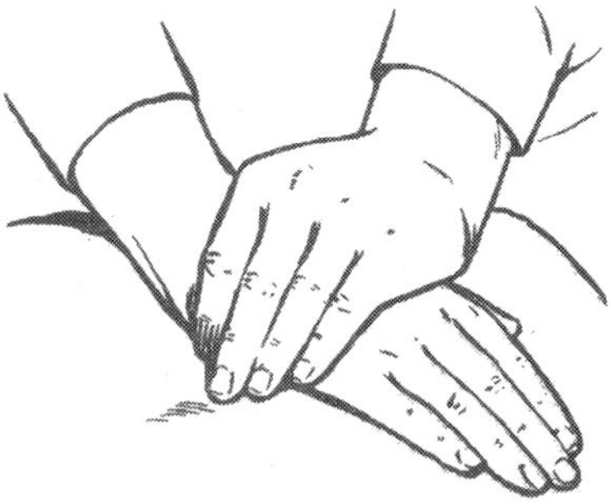

Massage and manipulation have been used since ancient times as remedial agents. Massage needs no description for the average reader, although the various methodologies can be as different as night and day. The application of the hands can range from a soft, sensual stroke to a penetrating pressure to a rhythmic percussion.

Manipulation has been vaguely described as the therapeutic application of manual pressure or force. This is fine, since manipulation can be applied to soft tissue and thereby becomes a form of, or outgrowth of, massage. Joint manipulation, in particular spinal manipulation, is another matter. It is defined as a "passive manual maneuver during which a three-joint complex is taken past the normal physiological range of movement without exceeding the anatomical boundary limit".

The defining characteristic of spinal manipulation for most people is the dynamic thrust, a sudden force that causes an audible release (cavitation, the "pop" sound) and is intended to increase a joint's range of motion.

This "popping" kind of maneuver, however, is only one of five grades of joint mobilization[4]. Each grade produces different effects by selective activation of mechanoreceptors in the joint:

Grades of Joint Mobilization

Grade I:

- Activates Type I mechanoreceptors that have a low threshold and respond to very small degrees of tension placed on the tissues
- Activates cutaneous mechanoreceptors
- If stimulation is oscillatory, will selectively activate rapidly adapting mechanoreceptors such as Meissner's and Pacinian corpuscles. (Examples: massage, Bowen Therapy, light Shiatsu, mechanical vibration)

Grade II:

- Similar to Grade I. (Examples: lymphatic drainage; Naturopathic "Bloodless Surgery" method)

Grade III:

- Similar to Grade II, but selectively activates an increasing number of muscle and joint mechanoreceptors as the tissues go into resistance, and less of the cutaneous mechanoreceptors as the slack of the subcutaneous tissues is taken up. (Example: deep tissue massage, Naprapathic soft tissue technic, Nimmo Technic, Neuromuscular Therapy, Shiatsu, Reflexology)

Grade IV:

- Similar to Grade III, but containing a more sustained movement at the end of range of motion, which is often near the resting or neutral position. This activates the static, slow-adapting Type I mechanoreceptors, whose resting discharge increases in proportion to the degree of change in joint capsule tension. (Example: Myofascial

---

[4] The term "mobilization" is today being used to describe passive range of motion as opposed to manipulation, but the traditional definition is being used here, as it has been used by naturopathic practitioners for the last century.

Release, passive range of motion, high amplitude/low velocity movement seen in Asian bodywork joint mobilizations, and Muscle Energy Technique)

Grade V:

- The classic high velocity, low amplitude (HVLA) thrust that is practically synonymous with spinal manipulation. The joint is positioned near to its end range of motion during this type of joint manipulation and an impulse applied to carry it just beyond[5]. (Examples: Osteopathic Manipulative Therapy, Chiropractic Manipulative Therapy, Naturopathic Manipulative Therapy, Oriental Medicine Manipulative Therapy, Japanese *Sekkotsu* Therapy)

Soft tissue manipulation is performed by a number of different types of massage therapists in the wide range of bodywork methods available. But it is also used by the physicians who are known for their joint manipulation, whom we discuss below. Many people do not associate this practice with naturopaths and Oriental medicine practitioners, but these two groups have also historically used these techniques. In the U.S., though, there are three specialties that have been associated in the public's mind with such methods since their first appearance as professions: Osteopathy, Chiropractic, and Naprapathy. Following is a brief description of the characteristics of these five approaches.

---

5 Although an alternate point of view has been expressed in recent years that a joint can be positioned near its resting or neutral position rather than near the end ROM, a position taken up by Evans and Breen in *A biomechanical model for mechanically efficient cavitation production during spinal manipulation: Prethrust position and the neutral zone.*; J Manipulative Physiol Ther 29 (1): 72–82.

Osteopathy

OSTEOPATHY: OSTEO (BONE) + PATHOS (SUFFERING) = DISEASE PROGRESSES FROM THE BONY STRUCTURE.

Osteopathy is a school of medicine was founded in the late 1800s by Andrew Taylor Still, a medical doctor whose insight prompted him to emphasize the musculoskeletal system in the belief that "structure governs function". The osteopathic viewpoint is that efficiency of the mechanical framework of the body regulates organic functions, and that harmony of the related parts depended on the way in which the musculoskeletal system operates. Dysfunction of the osseous and soft tissues at a given place, leading to dysfunction elsewhere by changing nerve impulse and blood supply, is traditionally referred to as a "lesion". Today, it is referred to as *somatic dysfunction.* Reducing that dysfunction is the purpose of the osteopathic manipulation.

Today osteopathic physicians are trained and licensed on the same level as medical doctors and the two function essentially the same[6]. However in philosophy, if not actual practice, the osteopath places emphasis on optimal body mechanics in regulating and maintaining health. Osteopathy has also adopted many soft tissue techniques, and those for visceral manipulation as well. Manipulative treatment is not performed by all osteopaths today but some practitioners offer it in addition to standard biomedical methods.

Chiropractic

CHIRO (HAND) + PRAKTIKOS (PRACTICE) = A LEARNED SKILL OF USING THE HANDS.

The second American manipulative discipline was founded by D.D. Palmer in 1895. Palmer had been an osteopathic student, but developed his own manipulative techniques. It

---

[6] An "osteopath" in the United Kingdom, however, is a practitioner limited to manual therapy.

is a system based on the diagnosis and manipulative treatment of misalignments of the joints, especially those of the spinal column, which are thought (as in original Osteopathy) to cause other disorders by affecting the nerves, muscles, and organs. Those misalignments are historically referred to as "subluxations" (much like the osteopathic "lesions").

Modern Chiropractic identifies what is now termed the *vertebral subluxation complex* (VSC) as the neural dysfunction that creates lowered sympathetic tone and changes in vasodilation that result in negative organic functioning. Malposition is still the chief criterion for manipulation. This can be determined by palpation or by radiographic imaging.

Note: Often a section of the spine is treated for "stimulating" or "inhibiting" effects—to speed up or slow down a visceral function. (As we will see in an upcoming chapter, the traditional acupuncturist uses needles to "tonify" or "sedate" points on the skin to the same effect).

Naprapathy

NAPRAVIT (CZECH FOR "TO CORRECT") + PATHOS (GREEK FOR SUFFERING)

Naprapathy was founded by Oakley Smith, a chiropractor, in the early 1900s. He developed a distinct set of techniques that differed from chiropractic methods, influenced by middle European manual therapies (hence, the Czech-derived name). He felt that the core of dysfunction was the restriction in the assembly of ligaments composing the bonds between the vertebrae. Subluxation theory was one of the main differences between Naprapathy and Chiropractic. Naprapathic principles declare that the fundamental problem to be treated with manipulation is the *ligatite*, a word originated by Dr. Oakley Smith to mean a pathological change in the overall tone of a ligament or its fibers at specific locations. Although the word is seldom used today, the resulting change in elasticity due to this type of lesion causes the spinal segments or articulations to change their positioning and relationships. Naprapathic manipulation is aimed primarily at soft tissue—muscle and fascia—but also creates repositioning of the bony structures as well. Loss of mobility, palpatory findings, and malposition are the criteria for manipulation. In recent years, Naprapathy has been referred to as *Neuromyology*. Doctors of Naprapathy (D.N.) or neuromyologists are only licensed in two states in the U.S. **Note: These methods are used to increase or decrease tonicity in the soft tissue as required.**

Oriental Medicine

Oriental medical principles state that the fundamental problem to be treated in manipulative therapy is a change in subtle bioelectrical energy flow through the tendino-muscular meridians (offshoots of the main acupuncture meridians that pass through the musculature). This is seen to be responsible for malposition of the joints. This is often due to a deficiency of "defensive energy" (*wei qi*), which normally circulates outside the meridians up to the skin level and is said to protect the body from external invasion. When this energy does not reach the cutaneous level, external elements such as wind, cold, dampness, etc., can penetrate the superficial zones of the body and there is a resultant excess energy in the pathways that make their way through the soft tissue of the musculoskeletal system. This results in myospasm and changes in ligament and/or tendon tone, leading to changes in the alignment of bony segments in the affected region. It is also recognized that such changes in alignment have adverse effects on the viscera due to the connections between reflex points along the spine and the internal organs. Treatment involves releasing trapped bioelectrical energy and supplementing it where necessary, then applying minimal manual pressure to reposition bony structures. A range of methods from Grade I to Grade V manipulations have historically been used. **Note: these manipulative methods are used in a context of reinforcing deficiencies and dispersing excesses in the tissues (once again, stimulation and inhibition).**

Naturopathy

NATURA (LATIN FOR NATURE) + PATHOS (GREEK FOR SUFFERING)

Although readily admitted to be a misnomer, the father of Naturopathy Benedict Lust used this term for his school of treatment encompassing all natural therapies. Since Homeopathy and Osteopathy were established bywords in alternatives to conventional medicine, the idea that nature could be used to eliminate suffering made the name acceptable.

Naturopathic principles declare that the fundamental problem to be treated in manipulative therapy is a change in soft tissue and interstitial fluid, which causes somatic dysfunction. Segmental malposition and loss of mobility, as well as spinal reflexes indicated for the illness under treatment, are the criteria for manipulation. In this way, the Naturopath frequently works backwards from the known organic pathology and finds the corresponding spinal manifestation (much like Spondylotherapy, covered in a later chapter).

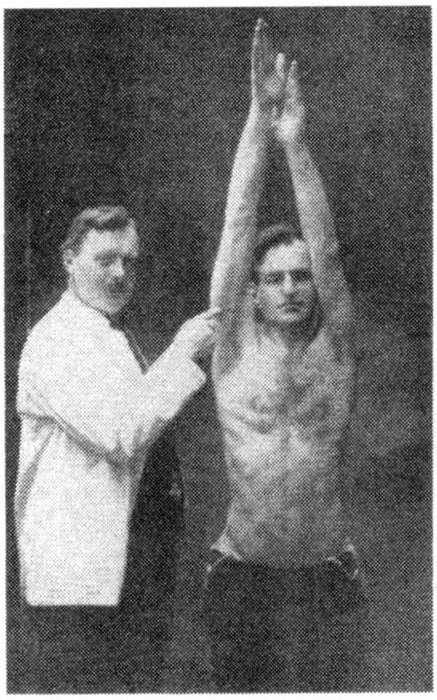

Frederick Collins, ND, DO, DC

Since early practitioners who gravitated to Naturopathy were chiropractors and osteopaths, the manipulative techniques that came to be taught in naturopathic colleges drew from these traditions. Earlier naturopathic students were taught to manipulate more like osteopaths but later programs have employed chiropractors to teach manual treatment. Naturopaths in England still have more of an osteopathic bent. Like osteopathic doctors eventually changed, only a minority of naturopathic doctors in the U.S. today use much manipulation in their practices.

Related to Naprapathy and later, to Bowen Therapy (covered in a later chapter), is the "Ligament Adjusting Technic" of Velma A. Rowley, DC. Originating in 1937, Dr. Rowley's approach echoed naprapathic principles but also presaged Bowen Therapy by several decades. Her success in treating arthritis by acting on soft tissue was remarkable, but today her work is largely unknown.

Dr. Rowley was a proponent of what she called "localized adjustment"; she applied chiropractic principles to the soft tissues. By delivering an impulse directly to the ligaments at problem sites (and not the bony structures), she was able to achieve results in rheumatism and arthritis cases that she had not previously achieved with standard chiropractic treatments. She would apply a rolling, flipping motion across the irritated ligament, and watched the joint re-align and inflammation subside. She wrote about her method in a national journal[7], but the method attracted little interest at the time.

Internal Effects of Manual Medicine

But aside from musculoskeletal problems, manual therapies are used to affect internal derangements with equal success. Just how does manual therapy affect organic processes? Although spoken nearly a century ago, this excerpt of a paper read by Chauncey Lawrence, D.O., before the North Carolina Osteopathic Society in 1918[8] is as eloquent as any we could provide today:

> When an osteopathic treatment is given, whether it be adjustment, stimulation, or inhibition, there is first *thigmotropism*, or response of the peripheral cells to touch. Then this impulse is carried over the nervous system and may cause motion of

---

[7] Rowley, Velma; *Ligament Adjusting*; Naturopath and Herald of Health, March 1941

[8] Lawrence, Chauncey, D.O., *The Biological Phase of an Osteopathic Treatment;* Journal of the American Osteopathic Association, 1918, Vol. 18, No. 4, pp. 170-172

> muscular fibers, say of blood-vessel walls, thus controlling the quantity of blood flowing to the region controlled by the nerve carrying the impulse. If carried to a gland there will be a secretion peculiar to the kind of gland, including the glands of internal secretion with their complicated and but meagerly understood influence upon the chemistry of the body.
>
> In case of a germ disease, the body, in accordance with the tropisms referred to, begins at once to elaborate antibodies in the blood to counteract the influence of the germ, thus establishing an immunity. These antibodies, of which antitoxin is an example, are chemical in nature just as the action of pepsin upon proteins in the presence of hydrochloric acid in the stomach is a chemical process.

Dr. Lawrence goes on to compare osteopathic treatment with serum treatment in infectious diseases. Since germs or their toxins are the antigen, and antitoxin is produced in response to them, inoculations have been historically used that are composed of antibodies raised in the bodies of laboratory animals, due to the problem of the disease organism often reproducing more rapidly than the human system can produce antibodies against it. The antibodies or antitoxin produced by the animal is used by the human body to assist in neutralizing the pathogenic organism. Dr. Lawrence points out that the formation of antitoxin or antibody is an example of chemotropism, or response to a chemical stimulus:

> Now, when these cases are cured by osteopathic treatment, instead of by using antitoxin, what is the explanation? Thigmotropism, or the response of the cells to touch during the treatment is transmitted to other cells and changed to

chemotropism, giving rise to the increase in the quantity of antitoxin produced, and these antibodies neutralize the toxin of the germ and the cure is effected. Notice, I do not say that osteopathic treatment calls forth any specific kind of antibodies. The germ already in the body determines the kind of antibodies produced, but the treatment causes the cells to elaborate more antibodies than would otherwise be formed.

Serum treatment deserves more success than its practical application has yielded. Unfortunately, there are two difficulties in the way. First, the serum of the horse is not identical to the serum of the patient, so the patient must react to the serum itself as well as to the antitoxin. Secondly, the virulence of the bacteria used in the animal is not the same as that of the bacteria in the patient, because bacteria are plants and the vitality of a plant differs with the medium in which it grows.

The osteopathic treatment does not have this two-fold handicap, for it works with the serum in the body of the patient and helps to form antibodies of exactly the specific kind to counteract the germ already in the body. Thus the treatment affects the chemistry of the body - another example of chemotropism.

If we place the fingers of both of our hands along the back of a patient in the mid-dorsal area and exert steady, deep pressure, we can soon observe gurgling in the stomach and intestines. What is taking place? The impulse has been not only transmitted from cell to cell through the nervous system, but also changed into peristaltic motion of the intestinal walls: an example of thigmotropism causing muscular action. In like manner glands may be caused to pour out their secretions. These secretions change the chemical nature of the lymph surrounding the cells and the cells reached by these secretions will respond to chemical stimulus. In this way the activity of the body cells is changed.

Or if the body has occasion to increase the number of white corpuscles in blood or to produce antibodies to combat disease germs, osteopathic treatment accelerates this functioning and so assists in overcoming disease. Furthermore, osteopathic treatment quickens the action of excretory organs so, as a combined result of these different responses to stimuli, a change in the chemistry of the body is effected. These are by no means the only results accomplished by treatment, but show only a phase of the work done. Then we conclude that thigmotropism or response to touch is converted into chemotropism, electropism, thermotropism, and indeed all tropisms, by osteopathic manipulations.

The opponents of manual medicine have pointed to the greater understanding of neurology since Andrew Taylor Still and D.D. Palmer's time, and have tried to portray chiropractors and osteopaths who manipulate as unscientific practitioners. Some criticisms of the original theories are not altogether unwarranted. For example, visceral functions depend on nerve impulses from a large number of common, but also different, nerves and plexi distributed widely; not on simple innervation by the spinal nerve trunks. The spinal nerves principally supply those parts of the body under conscious control, say the critics, and have little to do with visceral function, since organic performance is controlled by the sympathetic and parasympathetic nerves and not likely to be influenced by pressure on a spinal nerve. By this thinking one would assume that the critics' concerns were valid and that organic disease would not correspond to a deviation in the spinal column with pressure placed upon a nerve.

Nevertheless, autopsy studies have shown an amazing correspondence between the organic cause of death and a deviation in the spine exactly as described in the osteopathic and chiropractic charts. The collective experience of generations of osteopaths and chiropractors and their patients, not to mention the numerous clinical studies supporting osteopathic and chiropractic methods, show clearly that **spinal manipulation does produce demonstrable benefits, even if the original explanations for them are incomplete or flawed.** Regardless of mechanism of action, objective changes can be measured. With the reader's patience, I intend to build a case for a complex mechanism of action that unifies the various therapies described here.

3

THE MERIC SYSTEM

Chiropractic has long used the "meric" system as a means of defining locations for manipulation. The term means "pertaining to a *mere* (boundary)". The early chiropractors divided up the body into horizontal zones or bands, which contain several types of meres. A *vertemere*, therefore, is a zone defined by a certain vertebra or spinal segment and the tissues that are innervated the spinal nerves there. The influence of this spinal segment extends latitudinally around the thorax and influences internal organs and structures as well as muscular tissue. In fact, the various levels of influence have been given different names: Integumentary tissues in a particular zone are said to be the *dermamere*; bony tissue is the *ossomere.* There are as many meres in a zone as there are different tissues located at that level. Some of the zones overlap, which accounts for some variation among some neurological charts the reader may have seen.

While this terminology is not shared by other healing arts, it is worthy of mention in this book because it is the language used by the founders of Chiropractic to express some ideas that are of both historical and practical importance in our understanding of Uni-Syn.

As an example, the sixth zone consists of the sixth cervical vertebra, the pair of nerves superior to it, and all the tissue supplied with nerve impulses from them. Thus, the sixth *vertemere* influences the tissues of the neck, the Sternocleidomastoid muscle, the posterior portion of the mouth and pharynx, the thyroid, trachea, and cervical lymph nodes, the upper tissues of the bronchi, the superior portion of the shoulders, and the anterior portion of the arm surface, extending to the hand.

Chiropractic parlance evolved a number of generic titles for some of the major vertemeres; “M.C.P.”, meaning “middle cervical place” (3rd, 4th, and 5th cervicals), for example. Because its nerves affected the arms, the 1st thoracic vertebra’s vertemere was known as “arms place”, or “A.P.”. The region of the 2nd thoracic vertebra was known as “H.P.” (“heart place”) and was the target area for treatment in cardiac conditions. Similarly for the 3rd thoracic, known as “lung place”. This awkward terminology seems amateurish and simplistic today, but it has valid neurological underpinnings.

This is significant for the subject of this book, for this reason: The founder of Chiropractic, D.D. Palmer, established what became a standard treatment applied by chiropractors for decades after him. He referred to it as this simple directive: “Always adjust K.P., C.P., and Local.” This refers to “Kidney Place”, “Center Place” and Local (the zone or *mere* containing the affected organ or pain the patient was experiencing). Nearly all the early chiropractic textbooks, including Palmer's *Chiropractic Adjuster*, mention this method. Chiropractors in the early years considered this almost a commandment.

“Center Place” is the articulation of T5-T6, and “Kidney Place” is found at T11-T12. Palmer maintained that manipulation of these two spots created neurological effects that were global, or “constitutional”, as was sometimes used to express this idea in those days.

It is interesting to note that a completely different therapy, performed by a different type of practitioner, conformed to the same methodology as Palmer’s dictum. The naturopath O.G. Carroll, N.D. developed a simplified but powerful method of hydrotherapy in the first half of the Twentieth Century that he called “Constitutional Hydrotherapy”. This method is still taught in some naturopathic colleges.

Although the use of alternating hot and cold towels comes into play in other earlier hydro methods, what sets Carroll's version apart is the use of sine wave electrotherapy. In addition to the thermal effects of the water treatment, Carroll created a more dynamic general response by using electrotherapy at the same time. At two points in the procedure, sine wave electrodes are employed; first, at the level of T4-T6, then at T10-T12. "Local" treatment is also given, if required, by extra sine wave stimulation of an inflamed joint or affected muscle elsewhere, or on the abdomen if an internal organ was involved. Constitutional Hydrotherapy, therefore, derives some of its long-tested efficacy from the stimulation at "C.P., K.P., and local".

Bowen Therapy, as we shall see in another chapter, uses a foundation treatment with stimulation at the same "Center Place" and "Kidney Place" (although Bowen practitioners do not use these terms), with other regional movements as needed for the condition at hand, providing once again the "local" portion of the treatment as prescribed by D.D. Palmer.

Thoracic 1-2	Heart
Thoracic 3	Lung
Thoracic 4-5	Gall Bladder
Thoracic 6-8	Liver
Thoracic 7-8	Pancreas
Thoracic 7-11	Small Intestine
Thoracic 9	Adrenal
Thoracic 9-11	Kidney
Thoracic 12- Lumbar 1	Ileocecal Valve / Appendix
Lumbar 5	Uterus / Prostate

4

SOFT TISSUE MANIPULATIONS

The mechanical and chemical effects of the various massage methods on the human body need no discussion for the purposes of this book. Besides Swedish movement (which epitomizes the average person's vision of "massage"), there are many techniques that are concerned with more specific therapeutic goals; there are Trager Method, deep tissue massage, Zone Therapy (Reflexology), Hellerwork, Rolfing, Craniosacral Therapy, Feldenkrais, lymphatic drainage, and other specialties (such as Neuromuscular Technique and Myotherapy, which will be considered shortly). There are also Asian approaches to massage, which is more germane to our investigation at the moment.

The world of massage and the world of acupuncture meet in the Japanese tradition of Shiatsu. The term, meaning simply "finger pressure", belies its import. Shiatsu, in its most traditional form, could be said to be akin to acupuncture with the fingers instead of needles. It utilizes the same principles and points as acupuncture, and for that reason it is being singled out here because it relates strongly to the elements of Uni-Syn.

A Shiatsu session typically includes pressure on a series of points running along the spine. As we will see, the stimulation of reflexes adjacent to the spinal column is a factor in common with most of the therapies discussed in this book. Such overlapping is going to be dwelled upon repeatedly throughout these chapters because it is important for understanding how Uni-Syn's principles have been intuitively adopted by so many different approaches.

In Shiatsu, care is taken not only to press accurately on the spots that are indicated by the recipient's symptoms, or how the tissues feel to the therapist, but the *way* in which they are pressed (and for how long) also determine the effects. A light touch is used here, deep pressure there—according to whether there is a condition of *kyo* ("emptiness") or *jitsu*, ("fullness"). In acupuncture, a point that has excess bioelectrical energy is "sedated", while a point that is deficient ("empty") is "tonified". While the manipulation of the needle creates the needed action with acupuncture, the Shiatsu therapist uses his or her fingers to create either a stimulating or calming effect; different types of pressure and movement create differing actions. Superficial versus deep, stroking versus static pressure, pressing a series of points in one direction or the other—all create different effects within the body.

Another parameter for stimulating or inhibiting areas is the length of time the pressure is applied. Generally, a short duration *tonifies* or stimulates, while a longer application *sedates* or inhibits. This will be mentioned again in the chapter dealing with acupuncture, but is mentioned here first in order to point out that these twin actions of tonification and sedation relate to one of the three pillars of Uni-Syn: *Polarity*. While these therapeutic principles are well known and associated with Asian systems, most would not expect that they would apply to Western massage as well, and it received some unexpected confirmation in recent years. A study conducted at Los Angeles' Cedars-Sinai Hospital showed definite differences in the physiological responses to deep massage and light massage. The full story of this will be detailed in the chapter on the Minimization or "Less Is More" principle.

Neuromuscular Technique

Neuromuscular Technique (NMT) was developed by the famous English naturopaths Stanley Leif and Boris Chaitow. It is an offshoot of Nimmo Receptor-Tonus Technique, championed by American chiropractor Ray Nimmo.

Neuromuscular Technique is both an assessment method and a therapy. The fingers are used to sense changes in soft tissue by a light and perceptive pressure. The operator looks for sites of dysfunction, such as myofascial "trigger points" (discussed in the next section). Then deeper pressure is applied as a corrective measure, to overcome resistance of the more superficial tissues and stimulate the deeper connective tissues that are affected. The degree of pressure depends on the degree of resistance of the tissues. A distinctive sliding motion of the thumb and index finger is made during the assessment phase, which is peculiar to NMT. This characteristic will be brought up again in a later chapter.

Bloodless Surgery

A therapy used to great effect by many naturopathic doctors in the 1930s and 1940s was "Bloodless Surgery". Viennese physician Adolph Lorenz, MD performed many surgeries for congenital hip dislocation before abandoning the knife in 1892 for a soft tissue manipulative method, which became known as Bloodless Surgery. Applied to other conditions, it became a method that Lorenz taught in seminars after being brought to America to treat a special case. The orthodox medical community gradually became hostile, and Lorenz returned to Austria, but not before some prominent American naturopaths learned the method. Joe Shelby Riley, Paul Wendel, Harry Riley Spitler, and James McGinnis became proficient in Bloodless Surgery and taught it themselves, causing the technique to become a common tool in the naturopath's arsenal.

- Joe Shelby Riley, ND founded the National University of Therapeutics in Washington, DC.
- Paul Wendel, ND wrote a textbook[9] that was used in naturopathic colleges for years.
- Harry Riley Spitler, ND was the Dean of Central States College of Physiatrics in Ohio, and taught the method there, and at neighboring Metropolitan College.

---

[9] Bloodless Surgery: Technique With Treatment, 1945

- James F. McGinnis, DC, ND was a California chiropractor who became one of the best known bloodless surgeons to teach the method in the 1930s.

In this same time period, Major Bertrand DeJarnette was also practicing and teaching advanced methods of Bloodless Surgery. Dr. DeJarnette was also the developer of Sacro-Occipital Technique (SOT) in 1939, which is still practiced today by many chiropractors. He modified Bloodless Surgery technique to focus on reflex applications and referred pain patterns as diagnostic indicators of organic dysfunction. He taught throughout the 1940s and in the 1950s, his work matured with a decided emphasis on reflexes and their effects on the viscera.

By the 1960s, DeJarnette was still active and re-named his approach to Bloodless Surgery "Chiropractic Manipulative Reflex Technique" (CMRT). CMRT is a recognized technique in the chiropractic literature.

My mentor, Dr. Norman Abbe, studied both Spitler and DeJarnette's techniques of Bloodless Surgery, and the hand movements he showed me were at different times identical to Neuromuscular Therapy, and at others the same as Bowen Therapy movements (covered in an upcoming chapter). I have no idea now if this was due to two different sources of knowledge, but I am certain that the effects of all these techniques are the same, regardless of name.

Zone Therapy

Zone Therapy was developed by medical doctors William Fitzgerald and Edwin Bowers. Fitzgerald is believed to have learned a rudimentary version of this system from Native American healers. Zone Therapy was the first system known in the U.S. to make the claim that pressure applied to certain areas would create an anesthetic effect on distant areas. It not only eradicated the pain, but in many cases eliminated the root cause of the pain. Fitzgerald divided the body into five zones on each side of the midline, each beginning at the crown and running vertically down to the fingers and toes. Fitzgerald applied clamps, rubber bands, and other ligatures to these areas experimentally and produced anesthesia in other parts of the same zones.

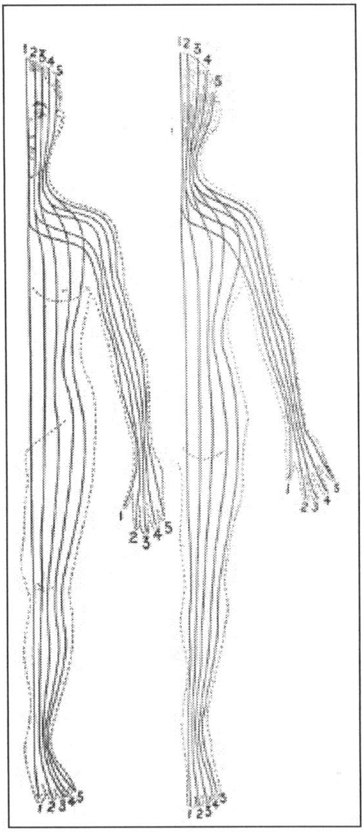

One principle of Zone Therapy stands out in the study of Uni-Syn: If a dysfunctional area cannot be treated directly, one can treat the same zone on the opposite side of the body with equally good results. Therefore, pain from a broken leg can be relieved by pressure on the other leg, in the same zone as the injury.

Joe Shelby Riley, ND studied under Fitzgerald and became a prominent expert. Zone Therapy became part of the curriculum in naturopathic schools after that time, and a student of Riley in the 1930s was Eunice Ingham, a nurse and physiotherapist who then concentrated on the feet and became the mother of Reflexology. Reflexology, the offshoot, has since eclipsed Zone Therapy in popularity.

Trigger Points and Myotherapy

Trigger points, a term originated by Travell[10] in 1942, are hyper-irritated spots in tense muscle tissue that often take the form of palpable nodules. They are clusters of cells in the muscle fibers that are believed to be locked in a dysfunctional cycle where blood flow has been reduced, and metabolic wastes are not being exchanged for oxygen and

---

[10] Janet Travell, M.D., personal physician to President Kennedy and researcher of myofascial pain syndromes.

nutrients. Biopsy examination has revealed that the points are excessively irritable and electrically active muscle spindles in the muscle tissue. If enough trigger points are located together, these form the "knots" that you feel when they are pressed. Compression of a point will cause local tenderness or referred pain. Trigger points often are not located in the area in which the person is experiencing symptoms, so it is a common experience that therapy applied to the area of pain is ineffective. Trigger points can be caused by injuries, stress, over use, nutritional problems, endocrine system dysfunction, and some diseases and infections.

Trigger points have several identifying characteristics:

- Compression of the point elicits local or referred pain;
- Rapid pressure, or needling of the tight muscle, can cause local twitching;
- Shortening of the involved muscle results in decreased ability to stretch the muscle, and pain in doing so;
- The muscle with trigger points can be weak but without obvious atrophy;
- The trigger point can be active (painful if moved), or latent (painful only if directly stimulated);
- Autonomic phenomena (such as increased perspiration or hair standing up) may be associated with activation of trigger points.

Trigger points are always tender to palpation and, although not all acupuncture points are tender, the points that are clinically relevant in a given case often are. Therefore, a trigger point can be an acupuncture point that is crying for treatment. Trigger points have been seen to appear where a branch of the local muscle's motor nerve inserts into the muscle and ends at a cluster of motor endplates. These sites contain sensory nerves of various sizes, and blood vessels with a close association to autonomic nerve fibers—making them by definition neurovascular points. Gunn[11] showed that such neurovascular points are correlated with the motor points of the body.

Massage therapists specializing in trigger points typically have training and specialization in Myotherapy, a focus on dysfunctions of the muscles and fascia. A myotherapist will examine posture to locate areas of derangement and to check for trigger points that may be causing referred pain to other areas. Various techniques are used to neutralize the sensitive areas. Manual pressure is most often used. Ultrasound and low level ("cold") lasers have been used to good effect also.

There is the poorly named practice of "dry needling", which is increasingly performed by physical therapists. This therapy is questionable not because of efficacy but because of the claim that the practice is not acupuncture—in spite of its being performed with acupuncture needles on acupuncture points. Acupuncturists have been needling what are now known as Golgi tendon bodies for a very long time. Apparently, proponents of "dry needling" feel that performing acupuncture while not calling it acupuncture, and using conventional anatomical rationale in place of Chinese meridian theory, places dry needling within their scope of practice. This is a controversy that is being argued in several states at present, with varying legal decisions.

A physician (such as a physiatrist) performing Trigger Point Therapy will typically inject the trigger points. Various solutions ranging from procaine to homeopathic medicines to simple saline solution have been used. Statistics show that there is little difference in what substance is injected. It is the action taken on the points that renders the therapeutic effect, which we would refer in Uni-Syn nomenclature as *Provocation.*

---

[11] Gunn C C, Ditchburn F G, King M H, and Renwick G J;. *Acupuncture Loci: A proposal for their Classification According to Their Relationship to Known Neural Structures.* American Journal of Chinese Medicine (1976) 4, 2: 183-195.

Soft Tissue, Old and New

Anyone familiar with Oriental medicine may have seen Gua Sha, the practice of scraping the surface of the body with dull-edged implements made of animal horn, shells, stone, or polished wood. Gua sha is often the treatment of choice for children, who would not tolerate having acupuncture needles in them for very long. Gua Sha increases blood microcirculation, which is obvious when one sees the extended erythema that follows a session. Lubricating oil is placed on the skin, and either long or short strokes are made with the narrow edge of the tool. In Chinese medical theory, this disperses "stagnant energy" in the soft tissue that promotes inflammation or is a byproduct of it. Gua Sha does appear to reduce inflammation and resolve soft tissue restrictions.

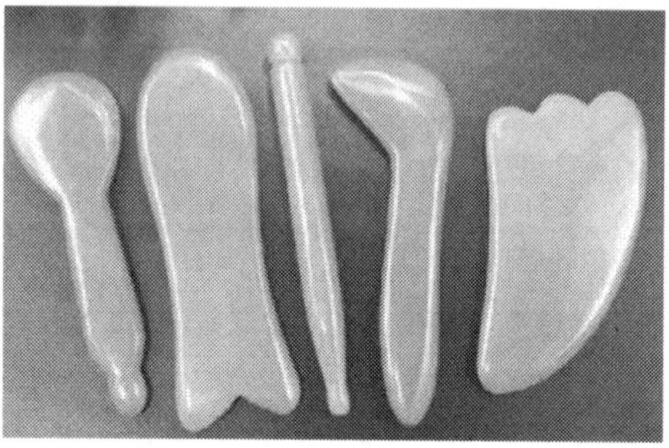

And, as with all things, a good idea never really goes away—it is just appropriated and re-named. While acupuncturists continue to use Gua Sha in their practices, other practitioners re-imagined the method in a more modern, "acceptable" form.

Without a trace of the trappings of the ancient Asian world and the mystical-sounding theories of acupuncture, Graston Technique® was given clinical trials at a hospital and has used this mantle of respectability to advance its popularity in the world of physical medicine. It is a modern offshoot of Gua Sha in that it utilizes a scraping action on the skin with various tools. While Chinese practices use natural materials for the instruments, this method uses stainless steel tools, shaped to fit various body parts. It addresses scar tissue formed by trauma, and restrictions in the fascia. Rehabilitation from injury is said to be faster and more

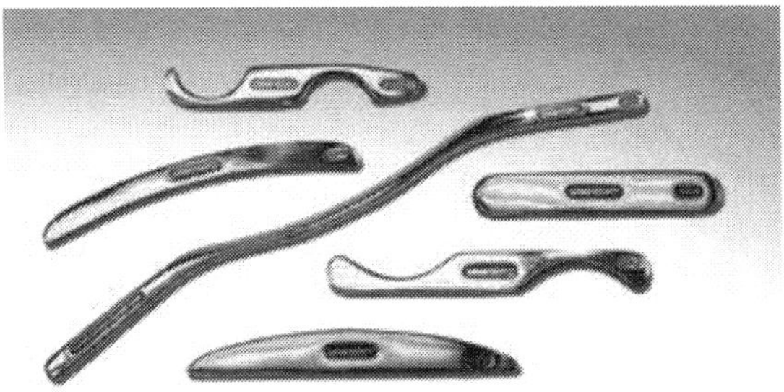

complete, with pain reduced and an increase in range of motion. A registered proprietary method, Graston Technique® is used by trained and certified chiropractors and physical therapists. And, of course, it has itself birthed imitators and variations.

In the professions that proudly claim to be "science-based"[12], there is now an officially-recognized subdivision of physical medicine called Instrument-Assisted Soft Tissue Mobilization; so "official" that it rates its own acronym (IASTM). The seemingly endless variety of methods like these owes its existence to the fact that sports medicine has become very big business. And because of the increasing number of practitioners tapping into that market who need continuing education credits, there is a burgeoning group of educators to put a new spin on an old method, which is also big business. This is not to suggest that the methods themselves are not worthy. This is mentioned because while those who are hard-nosed about scientific validity regarding some aspects of Uni-Syn simply because of some of the therapies we have discussed, they are likely seeing the modern, dressed-up versions as completely credible because of the "branding".

As has been pointed out previously, while the concepts behind some of manual therapies at the outset were not exactly aligned with modern science, the practices themselves were. Faulty theories about what was happening did not prevent it from happening. Much of the academic posturing today is to distract attention from the tried and true methods that are economical to learn and deliver, and replace them with approved, "science-based" versions.

---

12 A convenient way to distance oneself from the superstitious trappings of the Oriental medicine world, while doing almost exactly the same thing – because it works.

The scientific literature on soft tissue therapeutic systems at present seems to be skewed more in favor of mechanical explanations rather than neurological ones. However, one must consider that the subtle neurological signal being sent through the connective tissue to the brain, telling it to change neurological tone and allow the desired actions to occur, is one of the main mechanisms of Uni-Syn and indeed of the many methods we have reviewed. The relationship between the somatovisceral reflexes and viscerosomatic reflexes was addressed by older methods such as "Bloodless Surgery" in the 1930s and 1940s, and should not be lost.

But because of these methods being uniquely applied to musculoskeletal conditions, papers are not being written about the organic effects of soft tissue stimulation. It would be professional suicide, in fact, to assert that stimulation of the skin and fascia altered the internal physiology.

5

CHAPMAN'S REFLEXES

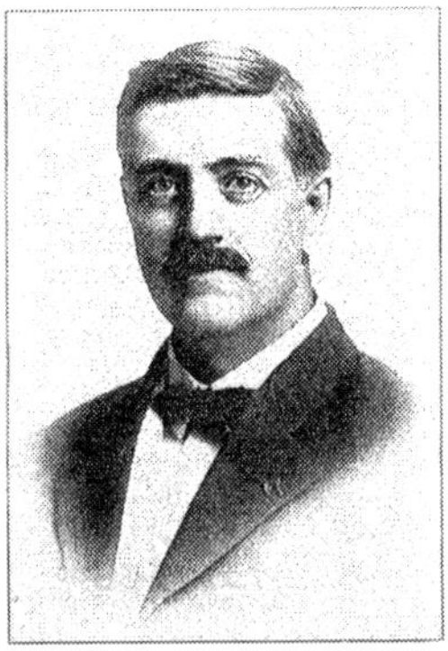

Frank Chapman D.O.

Chapman's reflexes were discovered by Frank Chapman, D.O. During his osteopathic practice in the early 20th Century, he noticed areas in the soft tissue that had a palpably different texture. He gradually realized that these were neurolymphatic reflex areas, and that they corresponded to specific viscera. Chapman was also able to make a correlation between these points and endocrinological functions, revealing them to be also neuroendocrine points, by today's understanding.

Chapman's reflexes are between the anterior and posterior fascia at specific points on the body, in the intercostal spaces. They feel tense when palpated. They are typically the size of a small bean, and are tender. For this last reason, they are diagnostic. They can be used for differential diagnosis of organic disease, as well as to regulate neurolymphatic communication to the affected organ.

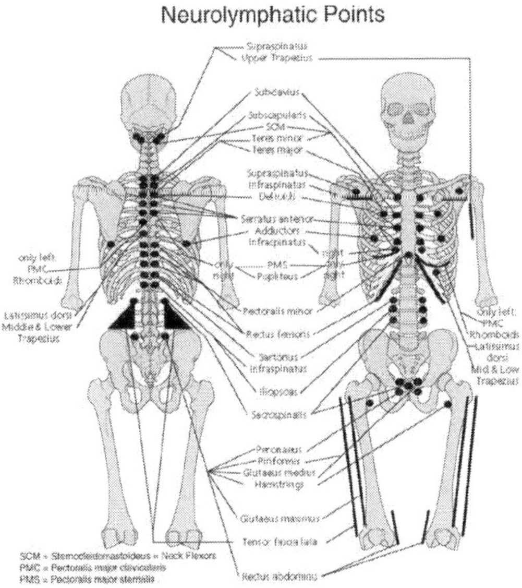

The technic is this: Make firm but gentle contact with the area to be treated with the pad of the finger. Make rotary motions while maintaining even pressure to "milk" the tissues of fluid and express it into the surrounding tissues. This reduces swelling, relieves the tenderness, and re-establishes a neurological "signal" to the affected viscera.

Chapman's reflexes are a similar phenomenon to what would come to be called *trigger points*, and are also what have been called *ah shi* points in acupuncture for centuries: tender spots that spontaneously appear when underlying tissues or organs are dysfunctional.

A number of protocols were developed for common ailments based on Chapman's findings. Manipulating osteopaths have used these for a century. An example would be the points Chapman found effective for laryngitis, seen here[13]. The superior surface of the second rib and the middle of the transverse processes of the second cervical vetebra. They are a quick, handy, and simple adjunct to any other therapy and produce rapid results.

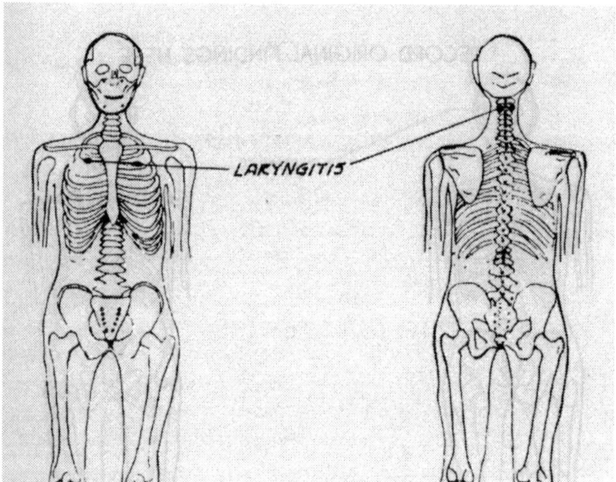

[13] From *An Endocrine Interpretation of Chapman's Reflexes,* Vol. 2, 1937 American Academy of Osteopathy

But note the correspondence of Chapman's spinal neurolymphatic points (left) with Hua Tuo's "vertebral points" of acupuncture (right), which will be discussed in an upcoming chapter.

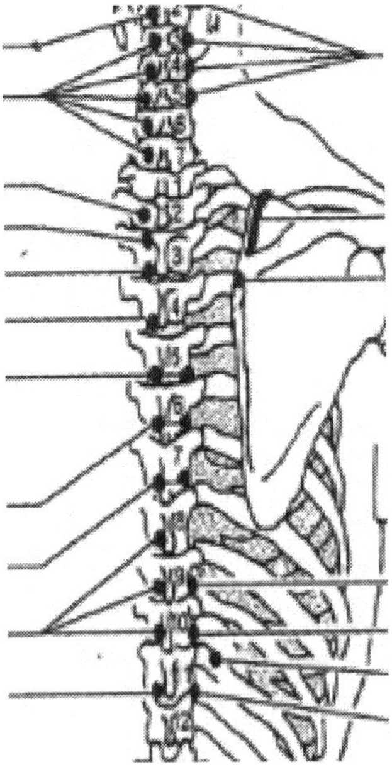

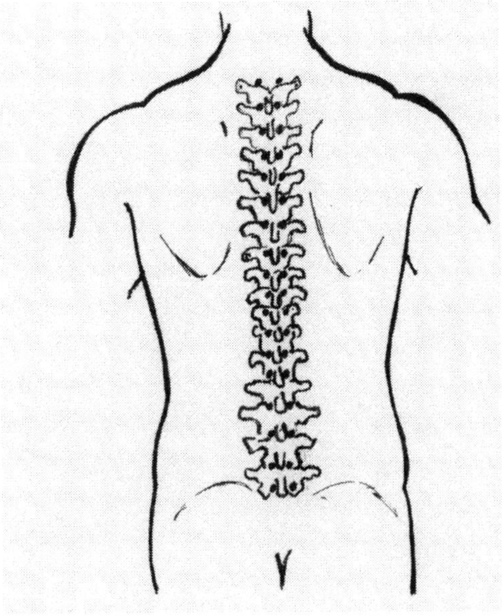

6

SPONDYLOTHERAPY

Spondylotherapy is a method of activating spinal reflexes without manipulating the spinal segments in the typical way. In the place of hand manipulation, percussion is instead applied to the spinous processes, using a reflex hammer (or a mechanical vibrator or concussor, or sometimes just the hand). The ulnar side of the hand proximal to the 5th MCP joint has been used effectively as a percussion tool, in a kind of "karate chop"[14].

Over 2500 years ago, the Chinese physician Mei Wei detailed the technic of tapping on the spinous processes to activate visceral responses and to treat musculoskeletal problems. The method established by him, we now know, was to stimulate the spine at the level of involvement (i.e., at the same dermatome as the pain site or the affected organ).

The affiliated spinal segment (or the affected spinous process) will typically be tender. Extremely tender points can be treated with a steady pressure, gradually increasing the poundage of the pressure to the patient's tolerance. Steady pressure is especially indicated in spasm.

Albert Abrams, M.D., officially developed and named Spondylotherapy as a way of eliciting spinal response with minimal intervention. There is evidence that his contemporary George Starr White, M.D. may have been the first to use this method, but he did not give the method a name. Later, Alva Emery Gregory, N.D., and Joe Shelby Riley, N.D., both elaborated on this technic for the

[14] A technic customarily called "hacking" in Swedish massage.

Naturopathic field. All four made contributions in the first third of the 20th Century to this simple method of treating the spine.

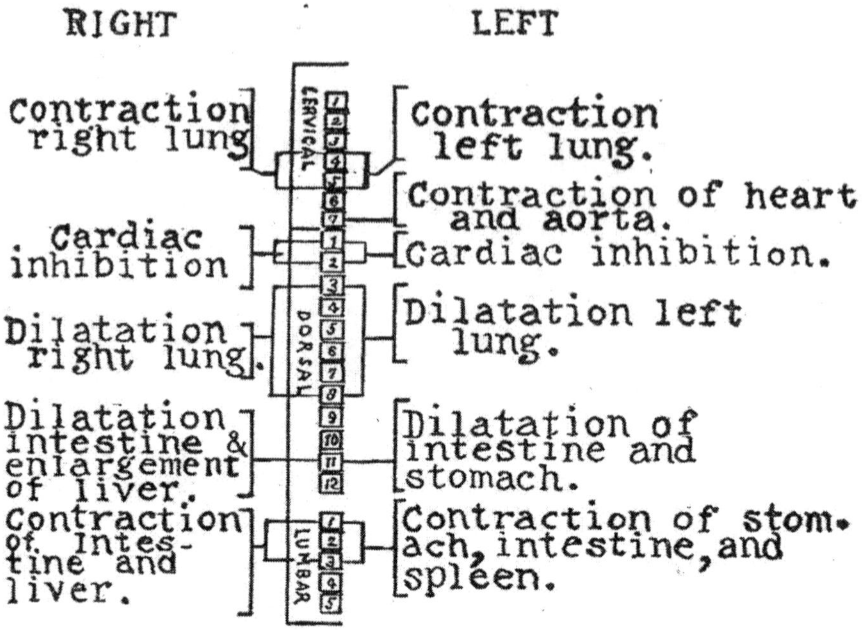

Visceral reflexes as elicited by firm pressure at specific sites on the spine. From Abrams' *Spondylotherapy* (Philopolis Press, 1918)

The amplitude of the percussive force and the length of time it is applied will vary according to whether the appropriate nerve needs to be stimulated or inhibited. This is a concept in common with acupuncture, in which one "tonifies" (stimulates) or "sedates" (inhibits) the points.

To stimulate a spinal reflex and increase the activity of the nerves (in cases of hypofunction and numbness, paralysis, etc.), a short duration tapping is applied; up to 10 or so strokes. Tapping is applied two strokes per second for the duration, then paused for 30 seconds or so to allow for the response of the nerve reflex, then repeated.

To inhibit the spinal reflex (in the case of hyperactivity or pain), a longer duration is used; but still no more than 25-30 strokes. Tapping is once again applied two strokes per second for the duration, then paused for 30 seconds or so to allow for the response of the nerve reflex, then repeated. In inhibition, sometimes a third course of concussion is given. In either case, the amplitude should be no more than 2-3 ounces of pressure.

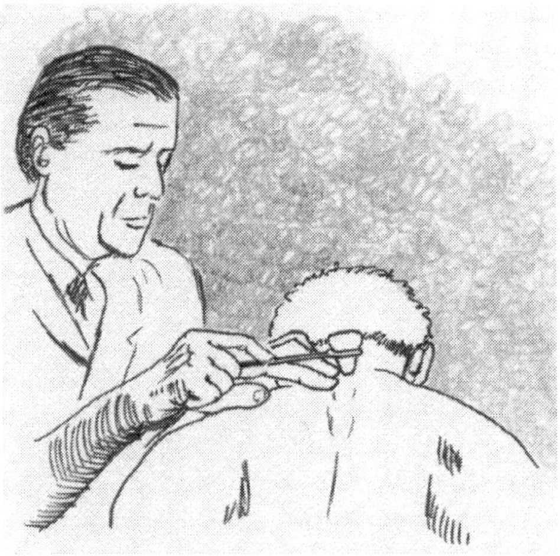

What should be pointed out here for its inclusion in the framework of Uni-Syn is that Spondylotherapy depends for its effects not just on the stimulation of the spinal column but on the *pause* between stimulations. This will be developed shortly.

DERMATOME MAP

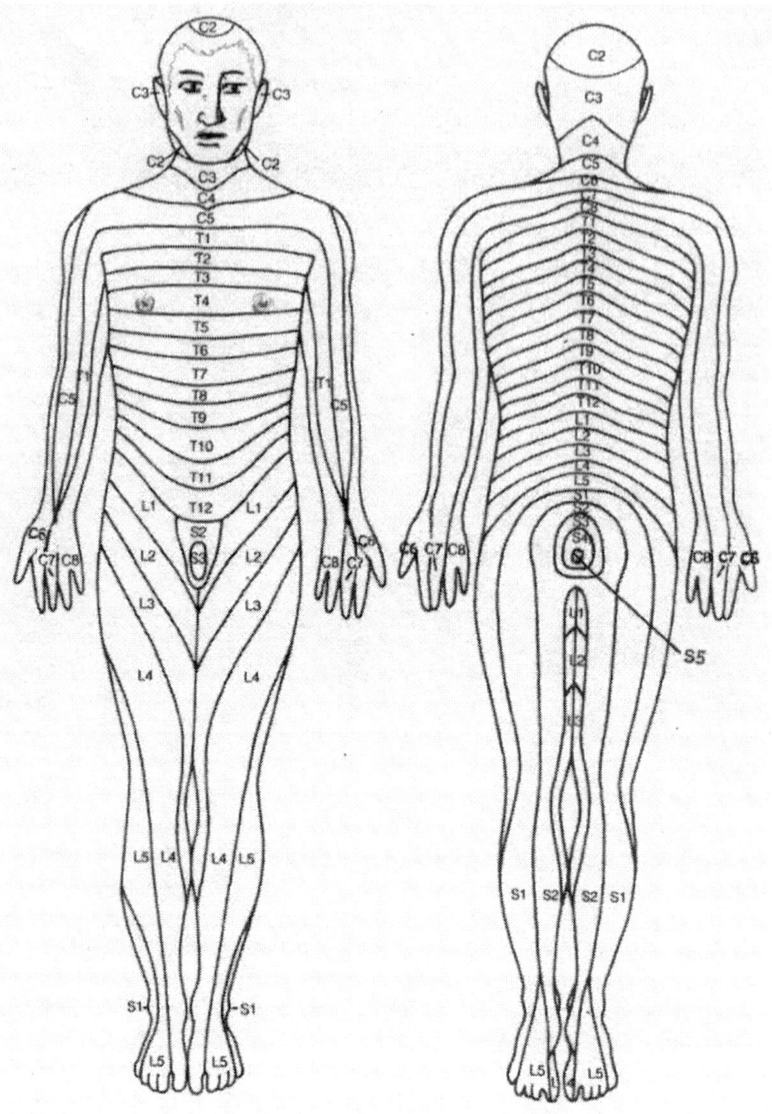

SPINAL REFLEX GUIDE

C1	Between occiput and spinous process of axis
C2	Middle of spinous process of axis
C3	End of spinous process of axis
C4	Spinous process of 3rd cervical vertebra
C5	Spinous process of 4th cervical vertebra
C6	Spinous process of 5th cervical vertebra
C7	Spinous process of 6th cervical vertebra
C8	Spinous process of 7th cervical vertebra
T1	Between 7th cervical vertebra and first thoracic spinous process
T2	Between spinous processes of 1st and 2nd thoracic vertebrae
T3	Between spinous processes of 2nd and 3rd thoracic vertebrae
T4	Spinous process of 3rd thoracic vertebra
T5	Spinous process of 4th thoracic vertebra
T6	Spinous process of 5th thoracic vertebra
T7	Between spinous processes of 5th and 6th thoracic vertebrae
T8	Between spinous processes of 6th and 7th thoracic vertebrae
T9	Spinous process of 7th thoracic vertebra
T10	Spinous process of 8th thoracic vertebra
T11	Between spinous processes of 9th and 10th thoracic vertebrae
T12	Spinous process of 11th thoracic vertebra
L1	Spinous process of 12th thoracic vertebra
L2	Between spinous processes of 1st and 2nd lumbar vertebrae
L3	Spinous process of 3rd lumbar vertebra
L4	Spinous process of 4th lumbar vertebra
L5	Spinous process of 5th lumbar vertebra

7

ACUPUNCTURE

Acupuncture is the most dramatic and well known modality in Oriental medicine, and everyone is familiar with the iconic rendering of acupuncture's central principle: the "Yin-Yang" symbol. One recognizes, after reading Chapter One, that this is an early depiction of the sine wave, and an expression of the concept of polarity. More profound than that, it points out that (in the language of the Chinese medical classics) "In the bosom of Yin, Yang is sleeping, and in the bosom of Yang, Yin is sleeping". So *the origin of a given polarity or force originates in its opposite*—very heady stuff, indeed.

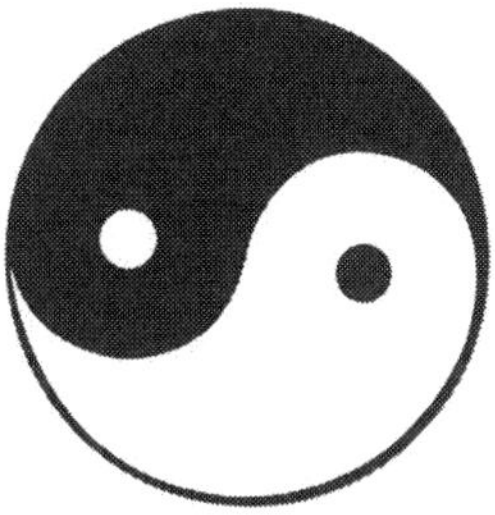

The Yin-Yang symbol signifies perfect harmony between opposites and represents the objective of treatment; that is, to restore balance by strengthening those functions that are too weak, and calming those that are too strong. The theory: Neurologically encoded information within minute electrical impulses travels along conductive pathways from the surface of the skin through various depths of tissues and reaches the target organ, maintaining a regulatory influence. Points along those pathways up-regulate or down-regulate those processes when stimulated in a certain way.

Tonification and *sedation* are the twin objectives for needling those points; tonifying where the signal is weak, sedating where it is too strong. This is not mere theory. Electrical resistance readings can be taken at points associated with the disorder in question and will be found to have a higher conductivity than other spots on the skin. After appropriate treatment, conductivity will be found to be closer to the median measurement. Conversely, low readings will be raised by tonifying stimulation.

There are various styles of acupuncture, with different emphasis and sometimes somewhat contradictory philosophies. The TCM or "Traditional Chinese Medicine" model from mainland China tends to predominate in the U.S. because it proliferated earlier and more aggressively than the others. I gravitated to a Japanese style of practice, but my early schooling was composed of Chinese/ Vietnamese teachings for the classical training, and German teachings for the modern part of our school's program. This was probably the first influence on my tendency to synthesize knowledge from many sources.

There are many different ways to render acupuncture. Rather than describe specific organized schools, I will just mention a few areas of emphasis, because there is significant overlap among all the varying approaches.

An acupuncturist could apply needles to:

- Distal points according to type of energetic dysfunction;
- Point combinations according to the diagnosis;
- Corresponding points on the anterior and posterior thorax;
- Reactive or tender points;
- Points along the spinal column;
- Points opposite the region under treatment;
- Micro-systems points, such as palm or ear points;
- Points according to the dysfunctional meridians;
- Points according to the diseased organ;
- A set combination of points for global effect;
- Only one or two points that have in common all needed actions.

Needling can be done at a depth and with a manipulation of the needle that causes a strong sensation. It is said in the ancient Chinese texts that when the energy arrives at the point, the sensation appears (called *deqi*). Yet, other practitioners (e.g.,*Toyo Hari* adherents) insert the needles very superficially, causing no sensation at all.

Such variation in practice is not unique; complete uniformity does not exist in other disciplines, either. Two chiropractors, for example, may be as different as night and day in their approaches. I wanted to give a fair representation to the field, though, before I endorsed any specific way to use this modality. I am also devoting a larger bit of space in this book to acupuncture, not simply because I am trained in its use, but because it is today the most heavily researched "alternative" medicine in this country, and that research establishes some of the foundations for Uni-Syn.

Scientific research on acupuncture in recent years has yielded much understanding of the role of the brain in explaining the pain-relieving and neuroregulatory effects of the ancient practice. Endogenous opioid-mediated mechanisms in the brain are used to explain the brilliant but mysterious successes of acupuncture treatment. Functional magnetic resonance imaging (fMRI) has been used to observe actions within the brain's "reward system" when needling is effectively done[15]. Changes in neurotransmitter activity and blood flow to the nerves, muscles, and skin have been verified. Segments of the brain controlling vision, for example, have been seen to light up under fMRI when a point on the leg traditionally corresponding to the eyes is stimulated. But these findings only partially explain the mechanism of acupuncture.

After much dismissal for decades by conventional physicians, science has verified that the points and meridians of acupuncture correspond to anatomical structures that have been observed with scientific instruments. Ions—electrically-charged particles—have been found to flow through ionic "stream beds" under the surface of the skin that coincide with the acupuncture meridians as long charted by the Chinese. These pathways of electrically-

---

[15] Tian He, et. al, *Neural Mechanisms of Acupuncture As Revealed By fMRI Studies*; Autonomic Neuroscience , Vol. 190, 2015; pp.1-9

conductive fluid have tunnels that reach the surface of the skin, called *Heine cylinders* and which have been found to correspond with the acupuncture points. Ions and electrons seem to be part of the flow of bio-electrical energy, or *qi* as it has been historically described. Yet it is not purely electrical in nature.

Photosensitive equipment has revealed that the acupuncture points actually emit light. A photon-releasing phenomenon is therefore present, and part of the multi-faceted mechanism of the transmission of information along the meridians.

Since the major acupuncture points appear to have an effect on endocrine receptor sites, it is reasonable to conclude that part of what has been attributed to the mysterious and vague *qi* is a hormonal mechanism.

In short: The effects of acupuncture, and the nature of the communication system called meridians, consist at various times and locations in the body as neural, peri-neural, hormonal, photonic, and probably other mechanisms that in pre-scientific times were lumped together under the collective concept of *qi*.

The Associated Points of the Bladder Meridian

The points of the urinary bladder meridian along its medial channel down the back (points UB-11 to UB-28) are often referred to as the *Associated Points* because of their reflex association with various organs, and are not (with the exception of one) associated with the urinary bladder itself. As one can see from the illustration, it is possible to treat somato-visceral complaints using acupuncture on these points along the back (or *acupuncture-like* provocation, with other types of superficial stimulation). When the Urinary Bladder Meridian was mapped out centuries ago, there was obviously already an observation that stimulation of these spots would affect organs other than the urinary bladder.

"Associated" Points of the Bladder Meridian[16]

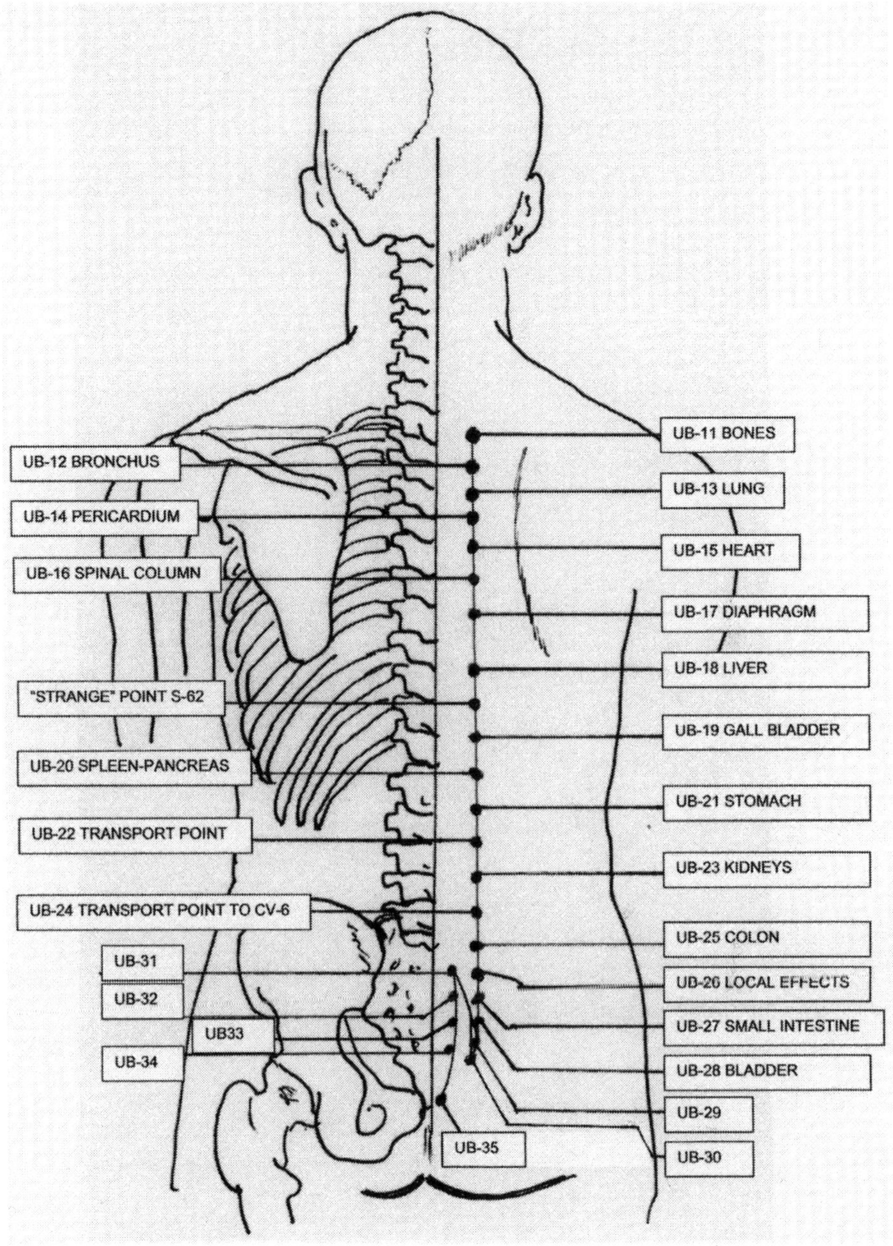

[16] Point 29 is typically used for lumbosacral pain. Points 30 through 35, while not traditionally grouped with the associated points, have applications in disorders of the ovaries, uterus, testes, and the urogenital system in general. Therefore, they do have organ correspondences.

The Vertebral Points

The Hua Tuo jiaiji points are a set of acupuncture points along the spine traditionally held to have been discovered by Hua Tuo, considered the "Father of Surgery" in Chinese medicine, among his other accomplishments. He was the first to perfom a colostomy, and reputedly the first surgeon to use anaesthesia, in China[17].

Hua Tuo's points (in modern terminology, the *vertebral points*) are located ½ *tsun* (half an "osteological inch", or acupuncture unit) from the midline along the spinal column. These bilateral points extend from the first cervical to the fourth sacral segments, although most practitioners utilize (and many textbooks list) only the seventeen pairs of points from T1 to L5.

Hua Tuo was the first to observe that somatovisceral complaints could be treated by points along the spine, rather than simply the *associated points* of the Urinary Bladder Meridian, or by points along the meridians that were associated with the problem organ or region. It was also recognized that pathological changes in the target organ would often produce a localized tenderness in the associated vertebral point. Therefore, the points are of diagnostic value as well.

To utilize the vertebral points is fairly simple: In order to treat any problem, the practitioner checks the corresponding nerve root for that organ and treats the points at that level of the spine.

---

[17] DeWoskin, Kenneth J., *Doctors, Diviners and Magicians of Ancient China: Biographies of Fang-Shih*; 1983 Columbia University Press.

Vertebral Points

The Vertebral Points lie under the skin over the intervertebral spaces and lateral to the spinous processes, approximately ½ "body inch", or osteological unit, from the midline. As mentioned, there are vertebral points along the cervical spine as well, but only the thoracolumbar points are displayed here.

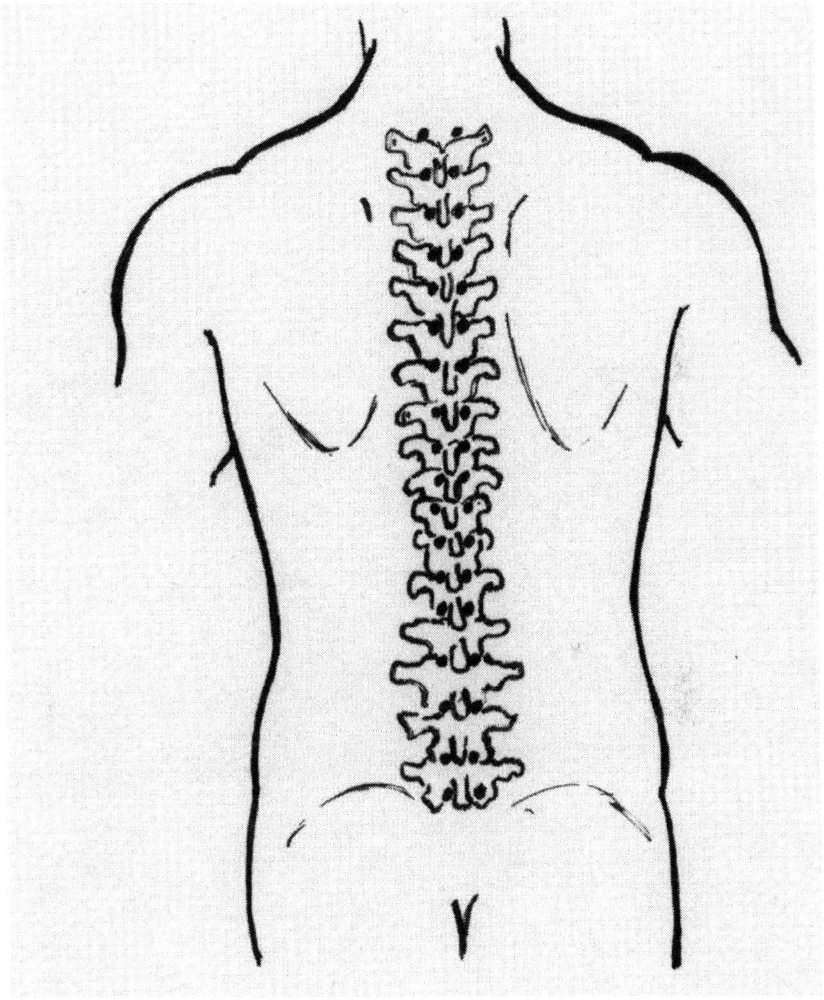

Relationship of the spinal column to Vertebral Points and Associated Points

Location is traditionally measured by "osteological inch" (width of the thumb at the widest part). The width of the index and middle fingers yields 1.5 units in breadth.

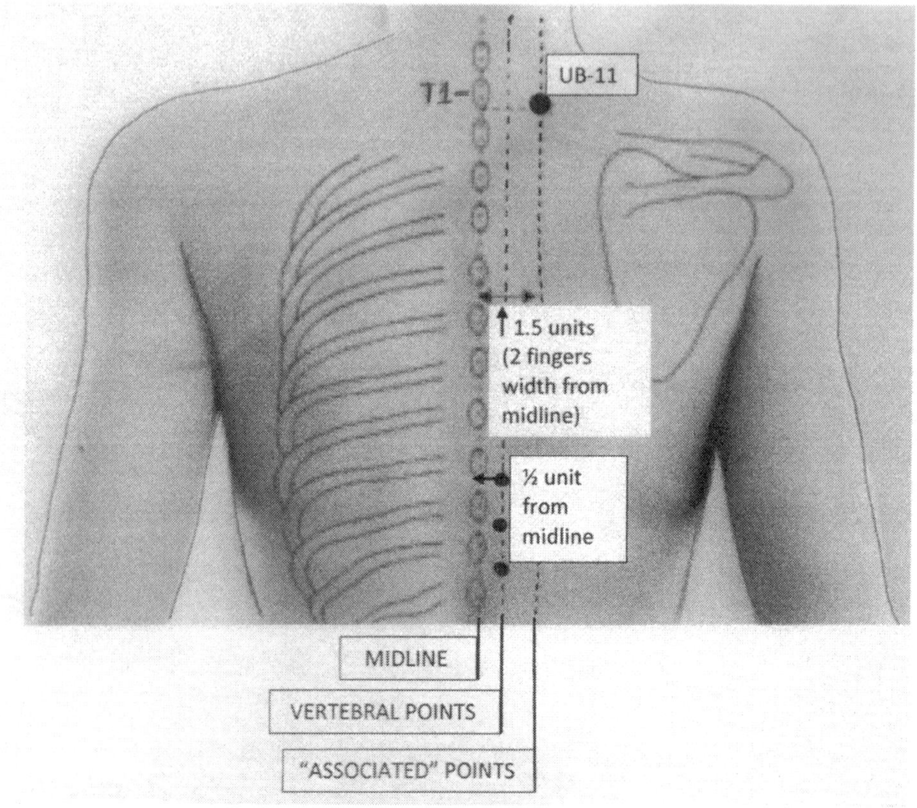

The relationship between the vertebral points and Chapman's neurolymphatic points, the *associated points* of the Urinary Bladder Meridian, and their visceral reflexes, and the "Meric Zones" of the Chiropractic spine/nerve/organ charts is self-evident.

It remained for a chiropractor and acupuncturist, Dr. John Amaro, to further elucidate the correspondences in Hua Tuo's points. Amaro, who may well be the Hua Tuo of his generation, observes a relationship between the vertebral points and the actions of points on the Kidney Meridian on the ventral surface of the body. Kidney points 11 to 21 are anatomically in the same place as Hua Tuo's points on the dorsal surface, although points 12 through 27 are more lateral to the midline. The kidney points apparently have a complementary action to the Hua Tuo points and can be used to further potentiate the actions of those vertebral points.

Amaro makes use of all the Kidney meridian points but has a novel innovation: He visualizes the Kidney Meridian to extend superiorly beyond where it is classically thought to terminate (subclavicularly), up to the level of the mandible and then posteriorly, to connect with the Hua Tuo point medial to point UB-10, at the level of C2 on the neck[18]. Thus, the Kidney meridian and the line of the vertebral points make one great Hua Tuo circuit, in Amaro's thinking, and serve as a very useful system of treating polar opposites.

Treatment appears to be more effective when complementary points on opposing sides of the body are treated. Dr. Amaro is a proponent of the Chinese *mu-shu* (front-back) methodology, and with good reason. His decades of successful clinical practice have shown extraordinary results with a wide variety of conditions.

---

[18] Amaro, J., *The Kidney Meridian and the Hua Tuo Jiaiji Points*; Acupuncture Today, January 2012, p.1

Whatever model is being used, it is undeniable that stimulation of acupuncture points produces visceral responses. But what are the mechanisms involved?

Manaka's "X-Signal"

The communications carried along the classical meridian network have been referred to as the "X-Signal" by Dr. Yoshio Manaka, a medical doctor who became one of Japan's foremost acupuncture researchers. Dr. Manaka hypothesized that there is a subtle "signaling" system operating at large in nature, which accounts for the meridian and *qi* concepts that have been described by the Chinese for thousands of years[19]. He theorized that this signaling system was the precursor of the more efficient and precise signaling systems of the nervous and endocrine systems, which developed later. The nervous system as we know it, which can be observed through evolution from lower-order to higher-order organisms, apparently replaced this primitive signaling system for the most part, because the neuro-endocrine system is a much more efficient signaling/ regulatory control system.

Manaka proposed that the older, more primitive signaling system, while playing an important role in lower order organisms (and in embryological development) began over time to be a less obvious regulator in the physiology of higher order organisms. Not quite a vestigial system (in the category of the appendix or the tailbone), it is still very important physiologically, but its operating levels are at such low levels of amplitude that it is barely perceptible. This makes it difficult to perceive, or to observe under experimental conditions. However, it is readily perceptible through its effects, for which the Chinese have been historically so talented in observing and cataloguing.

---

[19] Manaka Y, Itaya K., {1986). *Acupuncture as intervention in the biological information system (meridian treatment and the X-signal system)*. Journal of Acupuncture Society NY. 3-4:9-18.

An acupuncture point may have very specific effects within this signaling system, acting to switch the signals on or off, increasing or decreasing the amplitude, and applying the signal to a specific anatomical structure from a specific point. Manaka looked to some of the newest scientific theories and models (chaos theory, complexity theory, quantum mechanics) to elucidate his X-Signal model [20].

Needling Effects

Stimulating an acupuncture point can have three responses: A local reaction, a regional reaction, or a systemic or general reaction. Or, it may have no reaction at all, in which case the point chosen was not active at the time, was not accurately located, or insufficiently stimulated.

Local reactions change the electrical potential at the site of injury, modulating the presence of Substance P (the "pain chemical") by way of the attraction of opioid peptides, bradykinin, serotonin, and proteolytic enzymes, which have an anti-inflammatory effect.

Regional reactions have long been explained as occurring because of changes in the *qi* flow along the meridian connecting the adjacent tissue to the point stimulated. Since this involves two to three dermatomes, we now know that this occurs through a reflex arc of the stimulated nerves.

Systemic reactions produce the visceral changes that are central to acupuncture's ability to modify organic functioning, and this appears to occur through the central mechanism of homeostasis in the brain. Involved are cutaneo-visceral reflexes, viscero-cutaneous reflexes, cutaneo-muscular reflexes, musculo-cutaneous reflexes, viscero-muscular reflexes, Musculo-visceral reflexes, polysynaptic reflexes, and vegetative reflexes.

---

[20] Manaka, Y., Itaya, K., Birch, S., *Chasing the Dragon's Tail,* Paradigm Publications 1995

The neurochemical cascade caused by acupuncture, with brain neurotransmitter secretion, can account for the ability to modify acute and chronic pain, and also psychiatric conditions. To reduce the complex neurology involved by referring to it under the umbrella term *qi*, or "energy", is understandable considering the ancient history and cultural sources of the practice; however, this has been an impediment to its acceptance by establishment medicine—and also to its reliable usage, as we shall see.

Further, there are several additional factors in determining if a point is adequately stimulated. They are:

1. Area or point stimulated;
2. Combination of points stimulated;
3. Depth of insertion of needle, and
4. Intensity of stimulation.

Differing combinations of these four parameters will produce differing effects. This has been well delineated by Karanikiotes[21]. A brief description of these effects follows:

- Superficial needing stimulates the dermatomes;
- Very light needling (mild sensation) activates the autonomic nervous system and stimulates the viscerotomes;
- Deeper needling at the motor points stimulate the myotomes;
- Deep needling at periarticular points stimulate the sclerotomes;
- Very deep needling to the periosteum stimulates the osteotomes;
- Needling to a depth of 3-6 cm further stimulates the viscerotomes;
- Very deep needling with strong sensation stimulates the neurotomes.

---

[21] Karavis, M., *Neuroscience, Neurophysiology, and Acupuncture*, Web Journal of Acupuncture

Not only are different tissues affected by different types of stimulation, but different pathways are activated, due to the neurotome segments distributing nerves to different tissues from the same spinal trunk. A glance at the following illustration will show that the dermatome and myotome at a given location may stem from different spinal segments.

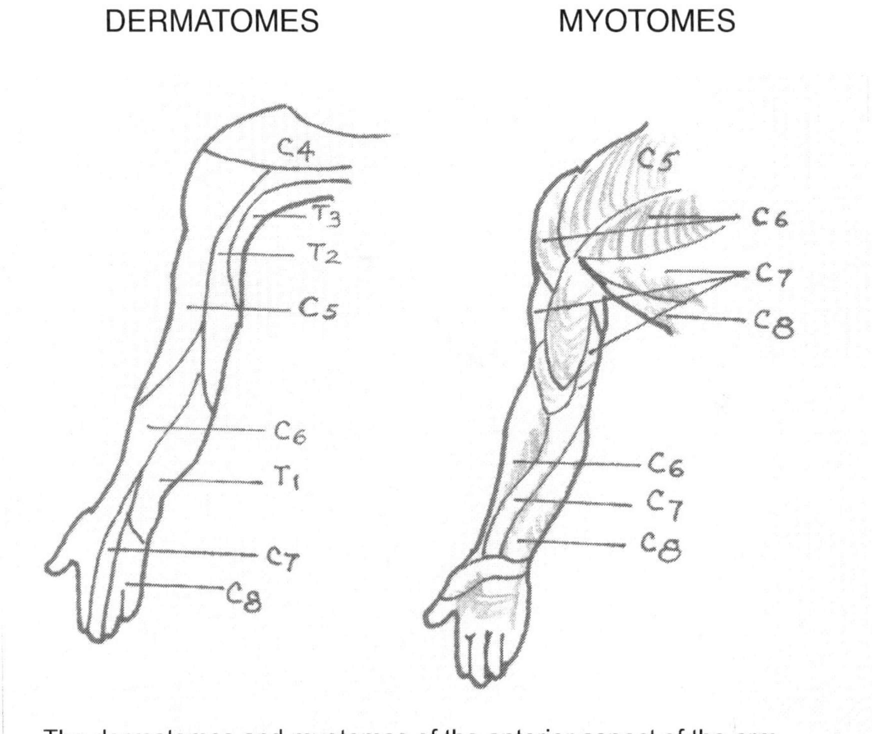

The dermatomes and myotomes of the anterior aspect of the arm

As one can see, different types of point stimulation produce different effects, and the success of a particular treatment is dependent on the practitioner deliberately (or accidentally, as is often the case) giving the body what it called for in that particular case. Classical acupuncture gives us indications of a specific set of points for a given set of diagnostic findings. It is incumbent upon the practitioner of effective acupuncture to determine in advance which level of action is needed (visceral, muscular, neural, etc.) in a particular treatment and properly select the appropriate points and stimulation strategy.

In addition, it should be determined which of those possible points will be amenable to treatment at that time, i.e., only "active" or responsive points will produce the wanted effects. This can be detected by electrical resistance measurement as previously described.

Acupuncturists who practice a narrow system, such as only using the "antique" or "five element" points, or only the anterior/posterior thorax points (*mu-shu* points), or only auricular points, will read this with dismay. Every methodology has its successes and failures. Effective practitioners of specialized systems, those who fit their patients to their chosen method, may be screening those who do not require the type of treatment they specialize in. However, the most successful practitioners are those who individualize their treatments and reach a larger and more varied patient population. In this regard, such acupuncturists are closer in philosophy to naturopaths, and naturopaths who utilize acupuncture tend to practice in this way.

Neural Therapy

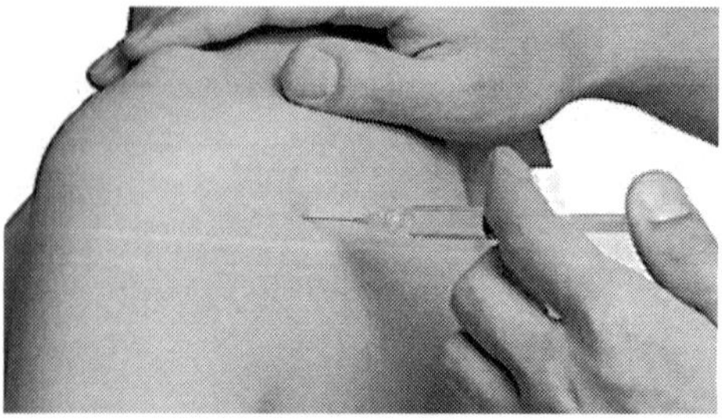

Another explanation for the effects of acupuncture comes in the form of Neural Therapy, a technic developed in Germany involving the injection of a local anesthetic (Procaine) into the appropriate areas. This method, pioneered by brother physicians Ferdinand and Walter Huneke, refers to these sites as *interference fields*. Any pathologically damaged tissue, or a local point with an abnormal electrical potential, acts as a stimulus to the autonomic nervous system. Neural Therapy corrects the dysfunction in the autonomic nervous system by stopping this interference field. In simple terms, it is acupuncture with the added element of a drug with its own chemical effects. It is estimated that 35% of all physicians in Germany use Neural Therapy[22].

The interference field is a modern explanation of the various types of "energy imbalances" described by classical acupuncturists: deficient *qi*, excess *qi*, blood or *qi* stagnation, etc. *No matter what terminology is being used, no matter what type of point stimulation is being used—the objective is to treat the foci of disturbance and remove interference fields.*

In the author's opinion, this should be the thrust of acupuncture treatment by the effective clinician. We should no longer have to rely on abstract theories because we have the means to evaluate the foci themselves (i.e., electrically measuring the points, thermographic measurement, etc.) and can use the same means to monitor response to treatment. Removal of the interference fields and correction of faulty autonomic steering is the result of accurate treatment, whether or not it is called "energy balancing", "harmonizing the *qi*", or other vague descriptions.

Venting Points

Most important in the removal of such interference is the use of what the author calls *venting points*. These are the most electrically conductive and clinically significant points in the region under treatment. Points said to be "open" points (that is, most effective for that time of day) typically display a reduced resistance to electrical currents; meaning that electrical conductivity is higher. Points that are connected with underlying inflammation do likewise. Such spots are typically more tender to palpation, though not always. They frequently display a change in temperature compared with the average temperature elsewhere on the skin. Therefore, palpation, galvanic skin measurement, infrared thermography, etc., can be used to isolate those points that

---

[22] One cannot imagine at the present time 35% of all American physicians using acupuncture!

are calling for stimulation. The "venting" action is the release of toxic metabolites, excess hormones, nerve pressure, lymphatic fluid congesting the tissues, and other obstacles in order to re-establish the orderly flow of *qi*, in the classical parlance.

The acupuncture points of major clinical significance all have proven neuroendocrine regulatory effects; and if one observes closely, they often are located exactly at motor end plates.

The acupuncture points of major clinical significance all have proven neuroendocrine regulatory effects; and if one observes closely, they often are located exactly at motor end plates, which makes acupuncture dovetail with physical therapy. The work of researcher C.Z. Hong[23] demonstrates this most clearly, and reinforces our position that many different disciplines recognize the practical use of the same anatomical truths; they just word it differently.

---

[23] Hong C Z and Torigoe Y ; *Electrophysiologic Characteristics of Localized Twitch Responses in Responsive Bands of Rabbit Skeletal Muscle Fibers.* Journal of Musculoskeletal Pain (1994) 2, 2: 17-43.

8

GENERAL NATUROPATHIC TONIC TREATMENT

In the 1920s, the prominent naturopathic doctor Frederick Collins used input from a number of other doctors who used manual therapies to develop a protocol for general use. He called it, variously, the Collins Universal Naturopathic Technique or the General Naturopathic Tonic Treatment. "Universal" in this sense is an archaic term meaning applicable to the entire body; what we today would refer to as having "global" or "multisystemic" effects.

Similar routines were used by osteopathic doctors (and Collins was also an osteopath).

(Patient lies prone)

1. Light thrusts are made in a caudal direction with the heel of the hand, to each spinous process from C7 to L1.
2. Light thrusts are made in a cephalic direction to each spinous process from L5 to L2.
3. Stand at left side, place right hand on the posterior iliac crest and left hand under patient's right acromion. Lift shoulder while pressing down on the iliac crest. Then switch hands to the patient's left side, pulling up on the shoulder with the left hand and pushing down on the iliac crest with the right.
4. Make contact with the heels of the palms on each side of the spine over the first ribs and make a light thrust obliquely toward the floor and toward patient's feet. Repeat for each rib up to the 10th rib. Then repeat in a cephalic direction, from the 10th to the 1st rib, opening up the articulations of the ribs in both directions.
5. From the left side, hook the right hand under the right anterior iliac crest and place the left hand on the right scapula. Press the scapula down while lifting the ilium. Move to the right side of patient and perform mirror image movements with the right hand stabilizing the

patient's left scapula and lifting the left ilium with your right hand.

6. Stretch the Sternocleidomastoid muscle by pressing the heel of the left hand against the area to the right of T1-T3. Using your right hand on the head, turn it to patient's left. Reverse hand positions and rotate patient's head to the right.
7. Apply the famous S-move (rotating the first two fingers or thumbs deeply in the muscle mass) on the laminae of the thoracic and lumbar spines.
8. Flex each leg once and push lower leg forcibly against the posterior thigh.
9. Place patient in supine position. Knead the abdomen from right lower quadrant to left lower quadrant, up ascending colon, across transverse colon, and down descending colon.
10. Stretch the abdominal muscles of each side by drawing up on the hip and pushing down just beneath the ribs.
11. Flex one knee and hip so that the thigh touches the abdomen, then rotate the hip in abduction and adduction. Repeat with the other leg.
12. Stretch the paracervical muscles, and perform a naturopathic manipulation of the neck.

The time required for a treatment: 5-7 minutes.

Pay particular attention to the instructions in Step 7 to **"Apply the famous S-move"** to the spine and keep this in mind when we cover Bowen Therapy in the next chapter.

9

BOWEN THERAPY

This manual therapy was codified in Australia in the 1950s by the originator, Thomas Ambrose Bowen. While it may appear to resemble other methods such as Neuromuscular Therapy, it is distinguishable by several characteristics. A Bowen Therapy session consists of several sets of gently rolling, cross-fiber connective tissue strokes, performed through the clothing in many cases. The basic Bowen movement distracts a muscle or tendon that is not under load and then rolls over it, without sliding on the skin. It is applied to the belly of a muscle, but also to the origin and insertion as well. There are frequent (and crucial) pauses between sets of movements, giving the body time to process the effects.

It is felt that the spindle cells and Golgi tendon bodies, which down-regulate the muscle's resting tone, are responsible for the relaxation of the musculature that occurs from the movements. The surrounding fascia decreases in density and becomes more elastic, allowing greater movement of blood and lymph through the tissue and enhancing nutrition to (and waste removal from) the site of injury. The action on the joint proprioceptors changes the recipient's postural positioning.

Because there is little skin stimulation, there is little distraction for the central nervous system and it focuses the brain's attention on the essential points (the limited number of precise movements also helps). A session is typically given only once every 7-10 days. The body continues to respond for several days afterwards, unless interrupted by injury or strong external stimulation (including new trauma, heat, and additional bodywork—even additional Bowen Therapy). Few sessions are needed in comparison to other similar manual methods (often as little as 2-5 sessions).

It is interesting to note that Tom Bowen's methodology was based on what he learned from a healer of some renown, Ernie Saunders, who used a "flicking" type of technique. Saunders had gone to the U.S. to learn from a Japanese manual therapist about whom little is known. Saunders returned to Australia and became famous for his techniques, which he taught to Bowen. It is likely that the Japanese practitioner was a Shiatsu master. Whether he was in turn influenced by Dr. Velma Rowley's "Ligament Adjusting Technique", is not known.

One interesting feature of Bowen Therapy is that, in cases of a one-sided or localized problem, the opposite or unaffected side is treated first. Recall that this strategy was present in Zone Therapy, and in one school of thought in acupuncture.

The core Bowen treatment utilizes a series of the rolling or "flicking" movements as previously described, in a sequence that stimulates several areas along the spine. Interestingly, they cover the "CP" ("Center Place") and "KP" ("Kidney Place") areas which the founder of Chiropractic said should always be treated.

Contemporary research into the Bowen method shows that the cross-fiber movement causes a piezoelectric effect that not only agitates restricted tissues into releasing, but that the neural network takes those sensory signals and re-distributes them as motor signals. When coupled with the requisite pauses between sets of stimulation, a deep response from the parasympathetic nerves sets in[24].

---

[24] Confirmed by heart rate variability (HRV) tests

It is interesting to compare the finger movement in "Bloodless Surgery" and that of Bowen Therapy, and also to consider the possible common actions below the surface of the skin.

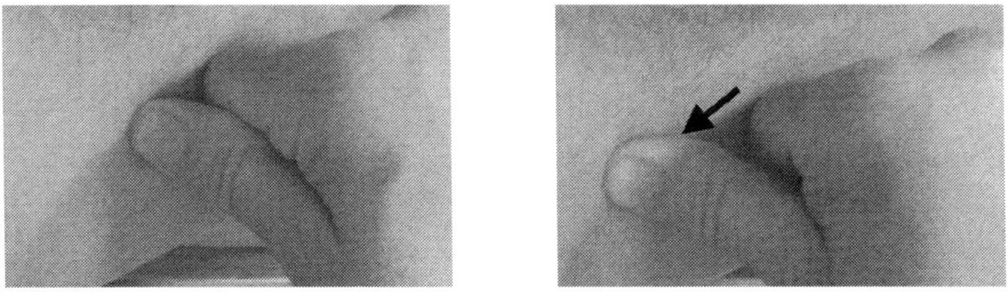

Bloodless Surgery anchors the tissue with the knuckle…the thumb stretches it.

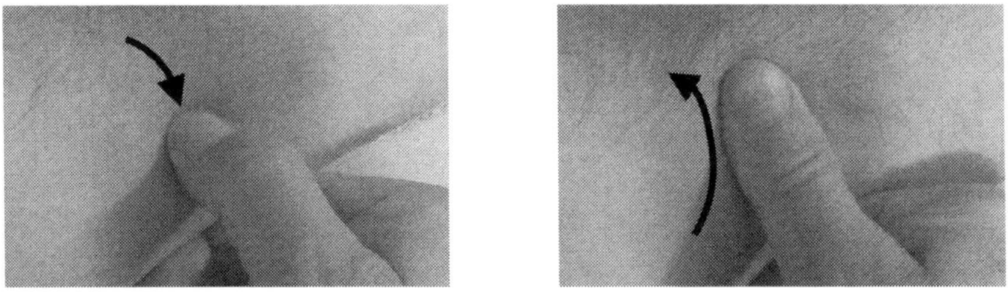

Bowen stretches the tissue in one direction…rolls back over the muscle.

While there are numerous explanations for the effects that are created by Bowen movements, there are actions that are somewhat overlooked: neurolymphatic and neurovascular responses, acupuncture-like effects, and even reactions that mirror the response to homeopathic medicines (as we will see shortly).

The rest periods are vital to the efficacy of Bowen Therapy, since they give the nervous system time to decipher, process, and respond to those sensory signals before relaying motor signals to the relevant areas and structures. Now we can see why treatment times with Spondylotherapy (covered in Chapter Six) are so short: **Reflex action coupled with a waiting period leads to the desired response.**

Once again, Japanese Shiatsu uses pressure along the laminae of the spine, just as the aforementioned Collins General Naturopathic Tonic Technique has spinal stimulation very much like Bowen. And, we have seen that Japanese-style acupuncture features needle insertion with a brief stimulation and then withdrawal, allowing the point to "rest" and the stimulation to be processed.

Bowen Therapy is said to create its actions by manipulating the superficial and deeper fascia. It should be pointed out that acupuncture points have been found to be small holes in the superficial fascia. While scientific research has never found any physical structure to the points (despite a concentration of nerve fibers and blood vessels enveloped in connective tissue—the aforementioned Heine cylinders), these small passages under the skin are significant because the Chinese word for an acupuncture point means "cave". These tiny perforations occur in 82% of the main acupuncture points, and the other 18% are located where there are other types of anatomical holes (bony foramens, etc.). Therefore, there is a connection between Bowen Therapy and acupuncture that has not been explored to any great extent in the literature before now. And the "famous S-move" referred to by Dr. Frederick Collins in his General Naturopathic Tonic Technique (covered in the last chapter) creates exactly the Bowen effect.

The rest periods are vital to the efficacy of Bowen Therapy, since they give the nervous system time to decipher, process, and respond to those sensory signals before relaying motor signals to the relevant areas and structures.

10

HOMEOPATHY

Since we have been focusing on manual therapies, it may seem odd to include a drug-prescribing methodology here, but in fact Homeopathy includes a very clear elucidation of the principles of Uni-Syn. If one wants to know how and when to apply a manual therapy (or any other therapy, for that matter) for the best results, one must have a grasp of the natural laws on which homeopathic medicine is based.

As you may know, Homeopathy "treats likes with likes"; that is, it uses medicines that mimic the symptoms of the disease in question. This is done because it was found that substances that cause a set of symptoms experimentally in a healthy person will reverse those same symptoms in a sick person. This theory was given more impetus after the observation that smallpox cases who were exposed to measles went into remission, due to the similarity of the eruption in both diseases. The measles seemed to cancel out the smallpox.

There are three main facets to homeopathic medicine:

- Totality of Symptoms: matching the complete symptom profile of the patient to the symptom profile of the remedy.
- The "Similimum": matching the symptoms of a medicine tested on healthy humans to the individual seeking treatment.
- The Minimum Dose: the least amount of medicine needed to effect the desired change.

This last aspect has been a thorny problem for Homeopathy, since it was found that medicines diluted beyond the capacity for chemical action will still act as a catalyst for healing. This provides ample claims of "quackery" by those hostile to homeopathic medicine. As far as this book is concerned, the matter of the "ultramolecular dose" is a non-issue. A medicine will work in *any* concentration, if it is the right medicine, and still be correctly termed "homeopathic". What is pertinent are the ways in which the principles of Homeopathy match up with the principles of Uni-Syn. To be succinct, we would all be better acupuncturists, chiropractors, osteopaths, etc., if we had homeopathic training—even if we never prescribed an oral medicine. This is because Homeopathy takes advantage of the same natural laws that Uni-Syn does.

For anyone desiring to apply Uni-Syn, it is essential to examine these points:

Newton's Third Law is important. Homeopaths were the first to find this physical law expressed in pharmacology, but it was ignored in allopathic pharmacology, until the work of Rudolph Arndt and Hugo Schultz. These two 19th Century doctors published a series of studies in which they proved that various chemical substances (arsenic, bromine, mercury, and iodine among them) had a stimulatory effect on cultures in low doses, but an inhibitory effect at higher doses. Higher doses still, and the cultures were killed. This became known as the **Arndt-Schultz Law**. It was not commonly discussed in allopathic medicine until 1944, when it was noted that while a large dose of penicillin would kill staphylococcus, a small dose would actually stimulate its growth. Then Arndt and Schultz's work was reproduced in 1960 in studies conducted and published by Townsend and Luckey[25], where a survey of conventional pharmacology yielded over one hundred substances that showed the same stimulation at low concentrations and inhibition at higher

---

[25] JAMA, 1960 May 7;173:44-8.

concentrations. They referred to this phenomenon as "hormoligosis".[26]

More simply rendered, this phenomenon is widely known today as the **bi-phasic dose response**.

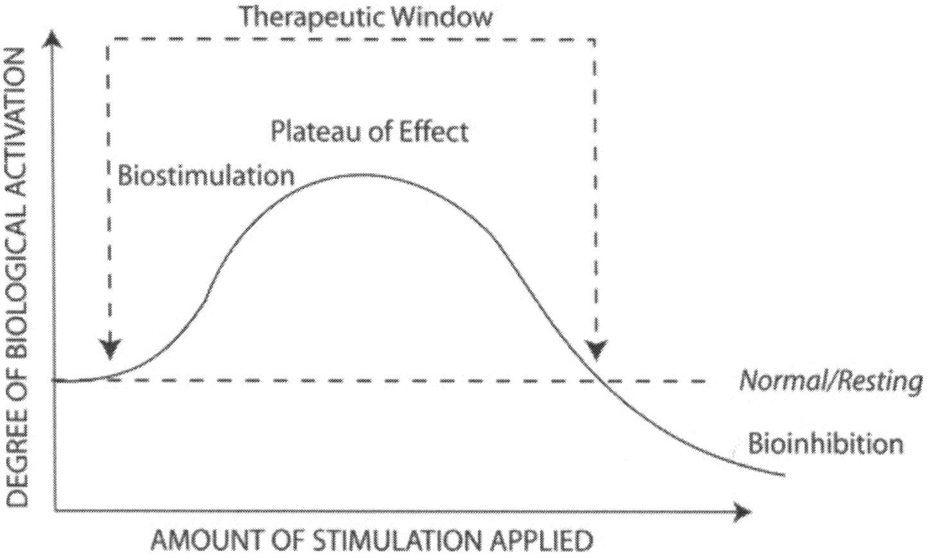

When discussing non-chemical forces, it is more tempting to invoke Newton's Third Law rather than Arndt-Schultz, but many biological functions in the human body are straightforward physical reactions and obey the same law. If you place an ice bag on the skin, it will initially cool the area. If left on, you will find that the area under the ice bag has become red and hot. You force the body to become cold, and it will respond by becoming hot. The fact is that the body will respond in an opposite way to how it is prodded. If one tries to down-regulate a function with medicine, the body will *increase* its attempts to produce the original condition. For this reason, tolerance to medicine is commonplace, and an increase in dosage is eventually necessary. Allopathic medicine seeks to overpower the disorder with an oppositely-acting force; homeopathic medicine prods it with a similar force, which the body then tries to reverse.

---

[26] This has been referred to as "hormesis" since 1982.

Similars repel or cancel. As we can see from the explanation above, a similar force will nudge the body to produce the wanted response. In Uni-Syn, we apply a force to the dysfunctional part that creates a message to the brain that the area is damaged. The brain then responds by sending repair messages to the tissues involved, *even though no actual new injury has been created.* This could be said to create a homeopathic effect without the use of an oral medicine.

Like poles repel and unlike poles attract.

Tonification and sedation effects can occur with different potencies of the same medicine. Polarity expresses itself in the various dilutions of homeopathic medicines. *Sarcodes,* homeopathic medicines made from organic extracts such as thyroid or liver, have differing effects depending on the degree of potentization. Low potencies tend to tonify the target organ, while higher potencies sedate. Therefore, a sluggish thyroid will benefit from a low potency while an hyperactive thyroid will benefit from a high potency.

Dose and wait. This dictum is the most important law in prescribing homeopathic medicines, and it perfectly expresses the importance of the waiting time in Bowen Therapy, the rest period after chiropractic treatment, etc. One does not repeat a homeopathic medicine until the previous dose has exhausted its action, because to do so will interfere and can bring to a standstill the body's response to the medicine. Likewise, in Bowen Therapy and Uni-Syn, one does not treat again until the healing response tapers off.

Lastly, Homeopathy—or at least an offshoot of it—contains one more facet that applies to Uni-Syn. This is the matter of the Weihe points.

The Weihe Points

In the early 1900s, a German doctor found correlations between illnesses and painful cutaneous points. Dr. Weihe knew nothing about acupuncture, but found tender spots that would spontaneously appear in a predictable fashion when there was clinical confirmation of a particular illness. He also noted that an appropriate homeopathic medicine would also predictably eliminate the tenderness. Since a large percentage of German physicians used homeopathic medicines, Dr. Weihe was familiar with the fact that homeopathic testing of substances often yielded specific symptoms. For example, test subjects who experienced the upper dose limit of *Nux vomica* developed a bruised soreness of the liver region. While this remedy is often administered for liver congestion, Dr. Weihe found that a point at the tip of the eleventh rib became tender when this medicine was indicated, and would normalize if he gave the medicine.

Acupuncturists will recognize this spot as the thirteenth point on the Liver Meridian, and it is palpated to assess hepatic function in Oriental medicine.

In 1904, German and French doctors Nebel and Jousset collaborated on determining the relationship between painful points and homeopathic remedies. The French homeopathic world was enthusiastic about this for some time, although the method was never endorsed in England, another hotbed of homeopathic practice.

The physician Soulie de Morant in France investigated Dr. Weihe's research and discovered a relationship to acupuncture, in which he was trained. Other French researchers found relationships between Weihe's points and homeopathic remedies: Rouy, Fourtier-Bernoville, Bonnet-Lemaire, Dano, Voisin, and DeLaFuye all contributed to Weihe's work.

This began a system of "body repertorization[27]". When the painful points were found by pressing on them, and the indicated remedy was given, the tenderness was reduced or eliminated entirely. This was almost always associated with a positive impact on the health problems of the subject, which confirmed the appropriateness of the remedy, *and* the reliability of the points to indicate not only the disease but the medicine.

Over time, more than 100 points were found on the trunk, neck, and head. Ten bilateral points on the head are used for differentiating 20 common remedies. 32 bilateral points on the thorax indicate a number of polycrests[28] and drainage remedies. The abdomen has 38 more points. There are also 25 vertebral and paravertebral points in this system.

This was a very exciting development, because it meant that when the clinical signs pointed to two or three homeopathic medicines, the doctor could differentiate between them by checking the points and seeing which was the painful, or most painful, one. It was also an aid in determining when to repeat or not repeat a dose, and the tenderness would return to the point when the remedy needed to be administered again. Since this is a common problem in daily practice, one would think that modern-day homeopaths would be interested in this.[29]

Dr. Roger De La Fuye, mentioned earlier, was also an acupuncturist, and he found that 153 of Dr. Weihe's points correspond to classical acupuncture points. The rest he designated "homeo-siniatrique". Much later, the same points were independently discovered in the Far East and are the newly-discovered points of the modern, scientifically-oriented

---

[27] Repertorization is the process of sorting through a large number of homeopathic medicines to filter out the ones that do not correspond perfectly to the case being analyzed.

[28] A broadly-acting remedy.

[29] Sadly, when I presented this material at a homeopathic case conference some years ago, I was disinvited from then on.

acupuncture. When I was in school, these were referred to variously as “new” points, “extra” points, and “strange” points.

A Doctor Margutti of Italy spent years finding correspondences between acupuncture points and homeopathic remedies which was very comprehensive—points will indicate one remedy in acute illness, another for chronic illness. Also he found cell salts and flower remedies that would also spontaneously reduce tenderness.

While work by Margutti and De La Fuye are influenced by their respective philosophies, Weihe’s discoveries stand out as empirical observations that stand the test of time.

A Sampling of Weihe Points

(As per Fortier-Bernoville, *Homeopathique Moderne No.6,* 1932)

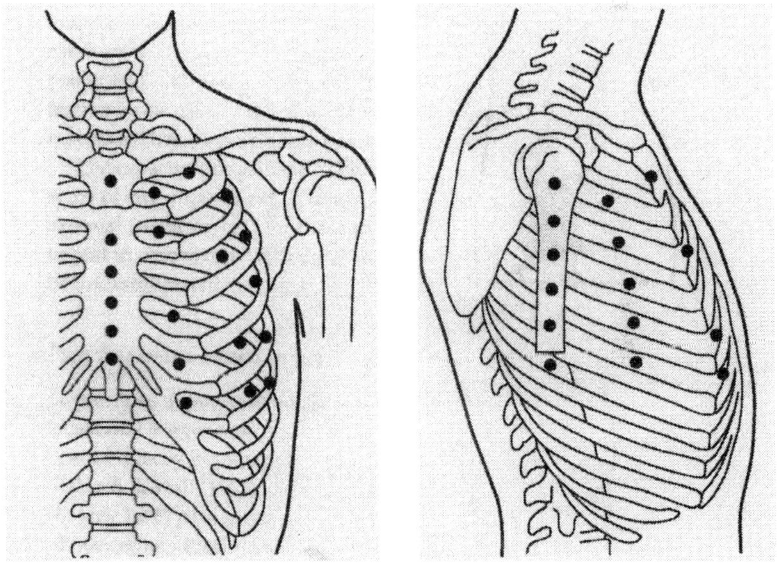

If you have read this far, you are likely to be fairly objective; but we remind the reader that homeopathic principles are not fanciful theory. There have been homeopathic hospitals all over the world, but in the United States, where it is an "alternative" with tremendous propaganda against it, the average person—even an intelligent person—will all too often view Homeopathy with suspicion or condescension.

It must be pointed out that homeopathic principles are actually used in "official", conventional medicine some of the time. Of course, the most obvious example of allopathic medicine using the "like treats like" idea is vaccination. Another is giving Ritalin, an amphetamine, to hyperactive children. Why would something that should make them more "hyper" make them more calm and focused instead? Conventional pharmacology explains it as a "paradoxical effect". It runs counter to the allopathic philosophy, but it works and so it is used.

A recent development is a better example of both the homeopathic methodology and the Uni-Syn principle of Polarity. Doctors at Johns Hopkins University have cured advanced prostate cancer by treating the patients with large quantities of testosterone. Usually, this hormone is *removed* in such cases, because it fuels the growth of cancer cells. They used extreme amounts of testosterone first, then used a drug that inhibited testosterone production. The shock of a large-scale reversal of the hormone caused the disappearance of the cancer cells. They call it "bipolar androgen therapy" (BAT).

This illustrates well the natural law that says that you can more easily reduce something if you first *add* to it—which is done with a homeopathic medicine that could cause the same symptoms of the illness (or a hormone that could feed the illness). But that natural law is also borne out by Uni-Syn treatment, where we will see that **adding to the brain's comprehension of the illness, dysfunction, or pain, we can induce cooperation in the brain to change the neural signals to the affected area.**

Not that the neural component is the only one, however. Using the Polarity principle can cause a cascade of biochemical reactions. A good example of this is a naturopathic method of hydrotherapy used in treating acute infection[30]. Immersing the patient in a tub of hot water, the head is covered with a cold compress and more hot water added periodically to increase the temperature of the tub. The patient remains for at least twenty minutes, during which time the pulse rate and temperature are monitored. The internal temperature increases (usually one degree for every ten pulse beats per minute) and an artificial fever is induced. After, the patient is bundled up and allowed to sweat (usually profusely) while resting. The procedure burns out infection, expels toxic waste, and strengthens immune response. Huge amounts of interferon are released in the body by this, just as in a regular fever, and antibody production increases twenty-fold. If fever was present before the bath, it "breaks" after because the purpose of the fever has been achieved. Once again, *adding* to the problem leads to a reversal of the problem, through the Law of Polarity (more in Chapter 13).

Homeopathic principles are actually used in "official", conventional medicine some of the time.

The Chiropractic method of Sacro-Occipital Technique developed by DeJarnette places padded blocks at critical places under the body to exaggerate the spinal dysfunction in the patient. This temporary increased distortion creates an opposite response in the subject's body. Likewise, Craniosacral Therapy takes the abnormal alignment of the cranial bones and "crowds" them, resulting in the body springing the segments back.

You can now see that it does not matter whether the treatment is manual, medicinal, physical, thermal, or electrical. Observing the predictable natural laws discussed here is what leads to success.

---

[30] The *Schlenz Bath.*

11

CONNECTIVE TISSUE, COLLAGEN, AND THE EXTRACELLULAR WORLD WITHIN

Research in recent years has illuminated electro-chemical processes in the human body in relation to a particular topic here and there. However, no one seems to want to draw from that knowledge to show how it applies across the board to procedures unrelated to their specialty. A synthesized view that unifies these disparate methods was needed. Ergo, Uni-Syn.

The manual therapies that we have covered here, in addition to acupuncture and some electrotherapy, now appear to all work through similar mechanisms, and all involving the peculiar properties of connective tissue and the extracellular fluids.

Once More, the Piezoelectric Effect

We gave a brief overview of piezoelectricity (literally meaning "pressure electricity") in Chapter One, and now is a proper time to better illustrate what happens in the self-lighting kitchen range or cigarette lighter, and why it has import.

A piston strikes the quartz crystal, producing a slight deformation of the material. This is referred to as "compression". Mechanical pressure or stress results in a displacement of ions within the mineral.

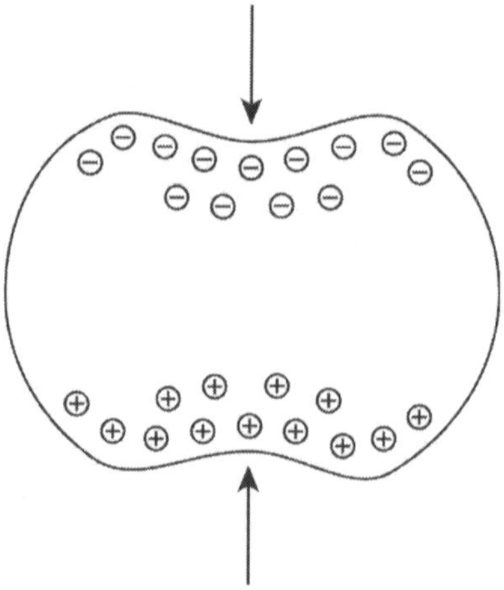

As seen, positive ions settle to one side of the material while negative ions line up at the opposite end. However, when the material springs back, they reverse positions. This is what produces the electric current, as the quartz (or other material) rebounds from the compression. This is referred to as "tension".

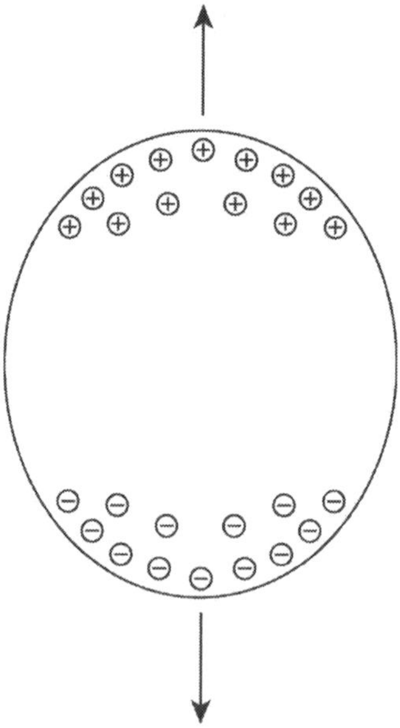

The flip from positive to negative and negative to positive will soon be seen by the reader as an expression of the Law of Polarity, as explained in the next chapter.

As mentioned in Chapter One, while quartz crystals are typically used in piezoelectric devices, other types of organic materials display piezoelectric properties. One of them is bone. Research has shown that this effect is due to *collagen.* Bone also contains apatite crystals, which are non-piezoelectric, but the properties of collagen display a structure that exhibits a semipermanent dipolar charge. Collagen is a dielectric material; that is, it conducts electricity despite acting as an insulator. Simply put, when collagen is stressed, it displaces charge-carriers that travel some distance—just like the quartz crystal that is stressed in the cigarette lighter or kitchen stove and makes a spark that jumps the gap to the gas and ignites it. This has been observed using piezo-response microscopy, and collagen fibrils predictably act as piezoelectric material.

This piezoelectric effect is thought to be a biological force sensor. The late 1970s and early 1980s was a fertile time for insight into this field as studies centered on bone resorption and re-growth were performed by top-flight researchers like Robert O. Becker, MD[31].

Please ponder the interrelationship between the different command centers in the brain (which have been shown to be activated by acupuncture) and the nervous system (modulated by Chiropractic), the vascular system (modulated by Osteopathy), the myofascial tissues (Naprapathy, Myotherapy, etc.), and the fluid component of the body, which is primarily water. The importance of water (the "memory" potential of water) to the concepts of Homeopathy is rapidly gaining recognition.

---

[31]Becker, Robert O; Marino, Andrew A (1982). Chapter 4: Electrical Properties of Biological Tissue (Piezoelectricity). *Electromagnetism & Life.* Albany, New York: State University of New York Press.

Causing the body fluids to change place rapidly is the effect of classical hydrotherapy, and one must admit that there are not only vascular responses to the application of water, but responses in the command centers of the brain, just as have been seen with acupuncture[32].

The movement of water throughout the tissues is not random; rather, it moves throughout a series of structures. The extracellular compartment extends throughout the superficial fascia of the whole body and small cylinders of this compartment project upward to the body surface. These projections are referred to as *Heine cylinders* and coincide with the majority of acupuncture points. German anatomist Heine determined that proteoglycans, blood vessels, nerves, sensory receptors, and muscles therefore constitute a functional unit, and interact[33]. The conclusion is that the acupuncture points are akin to little organs themselves. This, according to Heine, has implications involving the proteoglycan network beyond the generally accepted neurological and vascular functions.

The classical visualization of the acupuncture meridians upon which the points lie has been better verified in recent years. Anatomical research[34] by the Biomedical Physics Laboratory at Seoul National University, Korea, has shown fascinating corroboration of the ancient Chinese concepts. Staining with a DNA-specific dye, allowed visualization of ductwork[35] passing through the superficial fascia that appear to be synonymous with the meridians.

---

[32] Which explains the powerful systemic effects of a method like Carroll's *Constitutional Hydrotherapy*.

[33] Referenced in *Possible Applications for Fascial Anatomy and Fasciaology in Traditional Chinese Medicine,* (DOI: 10.1016/S2005-2901(10)60023-4)

[34] As reported in J Acupunct Meridian Stud 2009;2(2):93–106

[35] Referred to as *Bong Han Ducts*, or BHD.

Plenty of "programming" information can flow along the conductive collagen and fluid that travels from the brain through connective tissue to the surface of the skin, and back again. Whether the nodes or access points are seen as Bowen points, Weihe points, reflex points, or acupuncture points is immaterial.

In 2001, Dr. Helene Langevin of the University of Vermont reported in the Journal of the Federation of American Societies for Experimental Biology (FASEB)[36] that when needles were inserted and manipulated in known acupuncture points, a phenomenon her team called "needle grasp" occurred. It was found that connective tissue will wind around the acupuncture needle during manipulation, allowing the needle to pull and distort the surrounding tissue. This creates a mechanical signal at the cellular level, leading to distal effects that can activate cellular pathways, thus initiating healing.

Dr. Langevin's team found a stronger relationship between acupuncture points / meridians and the body's connective tissue than any previous research. In a statement that is quite outstanding for a mainstream biomedical journal, she writes:

> We propose that acupuncture needle manipulation produces cellular changes that propagate along connective tissue planes. These changes may occur no matter where the needle is placed, but may bc enhanced when the necdle is placed at acupuncture points."[37]

One of the most puzzling matters in bodywork of any kind is the phenomenon of tight muscles and dense fascial tissue "melting" when the appropriate technique is used.

---

36 Langevin JM, Churchill DL, Cipolla MJ, et al., *Mechanical Signaling Through Connective Tissue: A Mechanism For The Therapeutic Effect Of Acupuncture.* FASEB J 2001;15:2275-2282.

37 Langevin HM, Yandow JA., *Relationship Of Acupuncture Points And Meridians To Connective Tissue Points.* The Anatomical Record 2002;269:257-265.

Connective tissues are part of a vast internal real estate that contains a huge volume of fluid. The treatment that causes the tissues to soften brings about a process that has been called *solvation*. In one theory, the gel-like nature of the fluid is turned into a more water-like state by the solvation process. It does not seem to depend on purely mechanical force, as one might expect from compression, or the deep pressure of massage, or the dynamic thrusting of many manipulations. Subtle techniques involving light touch, or acupuncture, have created this effect also, as well as the soft tissue technics of Naprapathy.

This change in the fluid and consistency of tissue is seen to expedite the transmission of information throughout the entire network of connective tissue, which has fibrous systems throughout that may be a sort of semiconductor communication network. The collagen-containing fibers running through the spine, even through the intervertebral disks, can account for some of the far-reaching effects of spinal manipulation. Correction of alignment not only produces changes in nerve transmission but also semi-conductive impulses through the network of fibers that encircle any joint, not just the spine. Alignment of not only the bony structure of a joint, but alignment of this collagenous network could be the most important medium for changing the "programming" of the body's structure and function, and the underlying mechanism for such disparate therapies that differ in theory, objective, and methods.

This sheds light on the mechanism behind such "micro systems" as hand acupuncture and auricular acupuncture. The explanation of the embryonic formation of the "body map" on the ear sounds plausible, but why would the whole body be reflected on the hand? All the meridians do not run to the hand. It parts company with general acupuncture theory, but if we consider the role of connective tissue, which *does* in fact go to the hand, we now see just how every part of the body is communicating with every other part. This also solves an enduring conundrum for the acupuncturist as to why foot reflexology works, where again nothing in meridian theory can explain it.

Quoting Dr. Langevin's research one more time, she reports in a study of the of the arm[38] that "...more than 80% of acupuncture points and 50% of meridian intersections" appeared to coincide with inter- or intramuscular connective tissue planes. This solves another conundrum: The reason many medical researchers found that acupuncture at random spots seemed to create an effect, and therefore they felt this "de-bunked" the idea of points and meridians. However, in reality the connective tissue signal can be created anywhere, but more powerfully at the real points. Both factions are correct.

The Interstitium

The extracellular compartment previously described has been been under more scrutiny. It was discovered in recent years that the walls separating different types of structures like the fascia, veins, arteries, and skin were not solid barriers as previously believed. It has been found that they are actually spaces filled with fluid and simply supported by collagen. In 2018, the official anatomical name for these spaces was deemed the *Interstitium.* It is a network or "highway" of interconnected spaces through which a mucus-like gel flows, which binds with interstitial fluid. It is thought to be the source of lymph, and in this way is connected to the immune system. Researchers believe this explains the mechanism for some cancers migrating to other sites in the body.

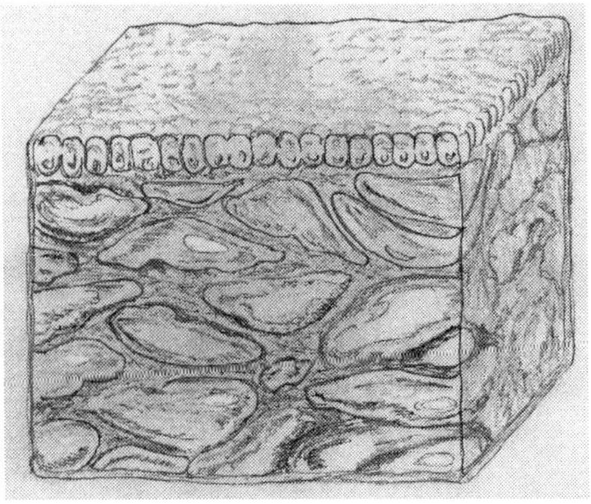

Interstitium

---

[38] *Ibid.*

Lymph channels pass through the fascia, and the action of the muscles extending and contracting pump it along and drain fluid and metabolic waste from organs as well as the musculoskeletal system. From there, it is returned to the vascular system. Obviously, the lymphatic channels need to be free-flowing to clear toxicity and to carry lymphocytes to fight infection.

Injuries to the fascia and other tissue cause a loss of pliability and even scarring, which inhibit the flow of lymph and interstitial fluid. Manual therapies such as massage, joint manipulation, acupuncture, and even hydrotherapy have been used for years to heal fascial or connective tissue dysfunction. All the systems built around manual medicine have long insisted that the musculoskeletal system affects organic function, which has brought them scorn by the mainstream medical profession. Current science proves this to be true, but the damage to their reputations is already too sweeping for their methods to be adopted by the dominant system of medicine.

Consider this:

- Acupuncturists still operate on the meridian theory and *qi* flow, long after neurological explanations for many of its effects have been established.
- Osteopathy was close to the truth with the concept of the osteopathic *lesion*, but finally embraced mainstream medical practice and de-emphasized manual medicine.
- Chiropractic remained drugless, but had to acknowledge other mechanisms than the correction of *subluxations* for the effects they create.
- Naturopathy has become increasingly modeled after mainstream medicine, with the move to prescribe drugs and perform minor surgery. Only a small percentage of naturopathic doctors today use any manual therapies, while virtually all doctors of earlier generations used them.
- Naprapathy alone, with its focus on connective tissue, had a model and explanation of action that fits today's understanding of the body.

Our current understanding of the extracellular matrix of connective tissue shows that **each school of thought was correct in its final assumptions even if incomplete in explaining the mechanisms by which it works.** The story of the blind men and the elephant was never more aptly applied. Naprapathy has been the closest to the truth, and ironically has the smallest number of practitioners.

SUMMATION

- Disease begins in the extracellular matrix of connective tissue.
- The connective tissue has gelatinous sugars, proteins, and electrically-conductive membranes that lie between the cells.
- The connective tissue is impacted by mechanical stress, and transfers that stress to organs.
- All musculoskeletal motions generate electric fields that are caused by the compression, deformation, and stretching of fascia, tendons, ligaments, and other collagen-based connective tissues. Like the nervous system, these messages spread throughout the surrounding tissues by way of conductive fluids and send information to other body parts.
- The network of connective tissue, called the *Interstitium*, therefore serves as a secondary nervous system.
- Therapies that reduce connective tissue dysfunction will restore correct information reaching the brain and normalize the information reaching the organs.

Uni-Syn is an attempt to define a reliable protocol for general use in manual treatment or in acupuncture (but can also apply to prescriptive treatment as well) that utilizes the mechanisms inherent in all the aforementioned therapies and maximizes them according to the natural laws that govern all of these therapies: Provocation, Polarity, Periodicity, Minimization, and Detachment.

To that end, we will cover each of these laws individually, beginning with the "Three Ps". At the conclusion of this book, we will illustrate a plan of action using these principles that any type of practitioner can use.

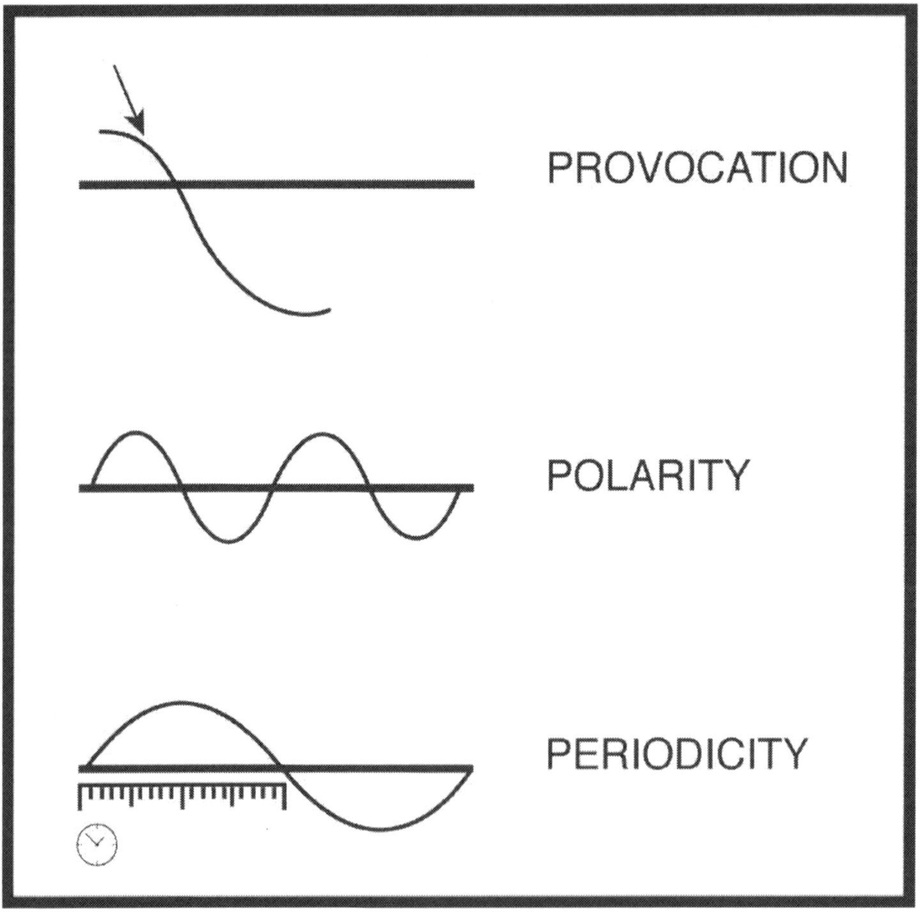

12

THE LAWS OF PROVOCATION

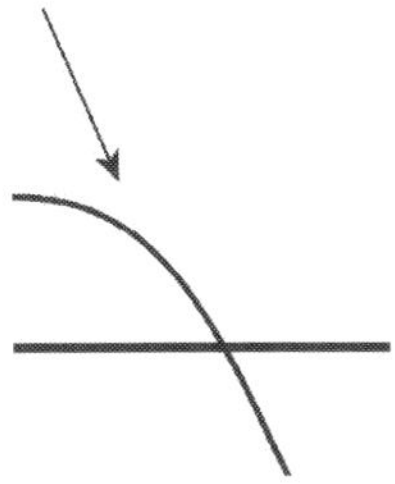

The principles and methods of tonification and sedation have been mentioned in several places up to this point. Although other terms are used in various disciplines for the same concepts—such as *stimulation* and *inhibition, reinforcing* and *reducing, augmenting* and *discharging, or* simply *light stimulation* and *heavy stimulation*—for our purposes any type of therapeutic action taken, internally or externally, will be referred to as **provocation**. To provoke a reaction, after all, is the objective. It is the body-mind system's innate capacity to heal that is being prodded by the therapy[39].

It is interesting to see the common thread running through the different therapies. Let us take a quick review:

- Acupuncture or acu-pressure is applied superficially to tonify, deeply to sedate.
- Finger pressure is light or stroking to tonify, and sustained and firm to sedate.
- Acupuncture needle insertion or acu-pressure is made when the patient exhales in order to tonify, and on inhalation in order to sedate.

---

[39] Of course, this is not the case when treatment is used, as in the dominant school of medicine, to override the body's natural responses. Suppression of fever with antipyretics, or suppression of reactions with steroids, etc., are used to restrain or contain the natural reactions, and therefore result in a damming up of the symptoms: If the treatment is discontinued, the problem is back with a vengeance.

• Chiropractic manipulation is often applied to a spinal segment to either "stimulate" (tonify) or "inhibit" (sedate) a process associated with that nerve trunk. Deep, sustained pressure is used to inhibit a hyperactive reflex, like the acupressure method.

• In hydrotherapy, application of water for a short duration, hot or cold, is "stimulating"; long hot or cold is "depressive".

• Galvanic current in the negative polarity tonifies, increases blood flow; in the positive polarity, it sedates, decreases congestion and blood flow.

• Sinusoidal current, while having dual polarity, can have polarity effects: Short use tonifies; long use sedates.

• In Homeopathic medicine, extended doses of a low-potency medicine are often given to "build up" or augment a weak patient's reactive ability, especially when there are degenerative tissue changes. A single dose of a high-potency medicine is given when the patient is strong enough to handle the cleansing reaction, a discharging of either physical or mental debris.

There are other examples, obviously, but it is enough to grasp the two different effects that provocation methods can cause.

Provocation Removes Interference Fields

In the chapter on acupuncture, we discussed interference fields briefly. Interference fields can be caused by endotoxins, exotoxins, or trauma. Whether something toxic penetrated the body from outside, or was generated from within, and whether that was caused by a physical or mental blow, the reaction of the body-mind system is rather predictable. Efforts are made to expel whatever noxious elements are causing the problem, and this observation is what made detoxification the major therapeutic goal in Naturopathy.

The fact that said toxins can cause electrical disturbances in the body in the form of interference fields bounces the ball right back to the acupuncturist, whose focus is the subtle neurological system.

But even the chiropractor, whose focus is supposedly the more gross neurological system, takes an action on these interference fields when the manipulation is done to best effect. Any chiropractic patient can tell stories of the powerful reactions that can be provoked by an adjustment. The same holds true, of course, for a manipulating osteopath, a naprapath, or a naturopath as well. Emotional releases during or after deep tissue massage are very common as well.

Provocation as a concept is not exclusively a therapeutic one. Injury *provokes* a response. Mental stressors *provoke* a reaction that can lead to emotional or physical decline. It is common to hear people say, "my nerves can't stand all the stimulation." We can picture the consequences. And when someone is melancholic, we say he or she is "depressed". In the first example, functions are turned up; in the second, they are turned down (or "down-regulated", in today's medical parlance).

The Body's Default Setting

Provocation, when performed as therapy, jogs the body-mind system into returning to its default programming. The default setting is health and healing[40]. The two components of that default programming, at its most basic, are *anabolism* and *catabolism.* Normal function and tone is maintained by the anabolic phase of taking up nutrients and building new tissue, and also the catabolic phase of eliminating waste and breaking down redundant tissue.

Provocation initiates anabolic activities—stimulation such as massage, manipulation, acupuncture, etc., results in a

---

[40] Illness being a deviation from the norm.

measurable increase in blood perfusion. With more blood bringing nutrients and oxygen into the tissues, repair is boosted.

At the same time, provocation initiates eliminative responses as well: the catabolic reaction of metabolic wastes being pumped out of the tissues, the increase in lymphatic drainage of the stimulated region, and the activation of the latent instinct on the part of the body to detoxify.

To illustrate this, consider the effect of an oral agent such as an extract of *Senna* or *Rheum* on the colon. Botanical medicines such as these, which stimulate the colon, result in an increase in volume and frequency of stool. Such stimulation does not produce constipation; instead it regulates the normal activity[41]. You say, "But those are laxative herbs." Yes, but they are laxatives because they are tonifying to the colon, and the colon's default programming is to regularly empty itself by peristaltic action. It is not the colon's instinct when stimulated to stop activity and hold onto its contents. It is an eliminative organ by nature.

Likewise, a kidney stimulant has a diuretic action, because that is what the kidneys do. Only a force that causes the kidneys to go against their default programming can slow down renal action.

But using examples of medication is distracting from our focus here and that is: clarifying just how stimulation applied to the surface of the body results in changes to organic functioning. This is the heart of Uni-Syn. To repeat what was stressed in the chapter on acupuncture: It is important to treat what the author calls "Venting Points", whether they are seen as active acupuncture points and/or *ah shi* points, trigger points, reflex points, or variations on vertemeres, Head's Zones, or whatever. Provocation applied to the Venting Points—whether by needle, finger, hand, a wooden probe, or an electrode—is a key part of Uni-Syn procedure.

---

[41] Too large a dose, of course, will *up-regulate* the organ and produce diarrhea.

As we discussed before, electrical resistance can build up in the tissues at various spots and partially block the transmission of the analog signal that directs the healing response. Trauma sites, in particular, are an obvious example. But scar tissue that has formed in the past is another area that frequently needs "venting"—many one-sided complaints are relieved by stimulating scar tissue in the opposite quadrant of the body.

Provocation Sets Polarity Effects in Motion

Provocation, whether by therapy, healthy stimulation, or by injury or disease-inducing factors, causes polarity effects. Polarity will be discussed in detail in the next chapter, but this will serve as an introduction.

The internal programming of the human being has been unchanged since ancient times with regards to psychology and physiology. Threats to our safety and well-being cause internal chemical reactions that lead ultimately to violence. Once the violent action is consummated, there is a release of the emotions that led to it, and there is a rest/relaxation phase that follows.

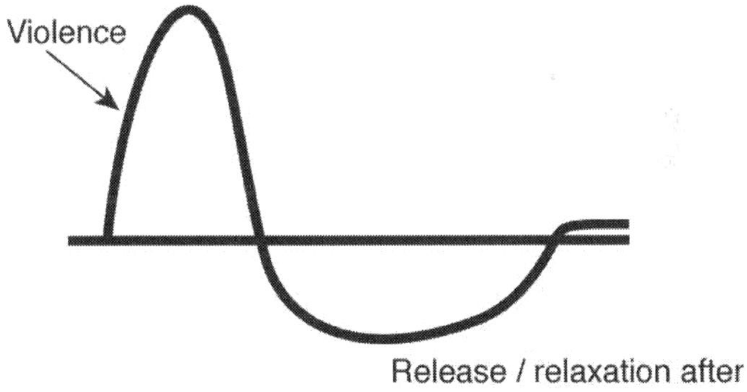

Now in our modern society, not only are there a multitude of stress-inducing factors on a daily basis, but violence is not appropriate for most of them, and there are rules that prevent a violent resolution of those problems in any case. So in a world where we cannot run away from stress, we simultaneously have no release of those chemical manifestations of the stress[42]. There is no option to alleviate these effects through physical violence, which for thousands of years has been the instinctive solution. This leads to a "no release" situation when seen from a polarity perspective:

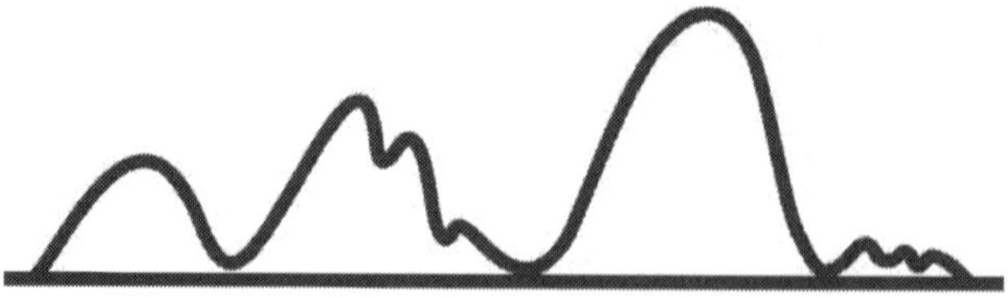

No release

The repeated stimulation in the positive phase causes chemical reactions involving Interleukin 6, TNF receptor 2, etc. Inflammatory proteins thus generated can cause any combination of health problems. But they are not counterbalanced by a release phase where endorphins, enkephalins, and other brain chemicals come to the rescue. So the inflammatory effects accumulate and result in disease states. It is no oversimplification to say that stress is the ultimate cause of disease, if one takes into consideration that microorganisms can also cause the same internal responses as circumstantial stresses. Germ Theory notwithstanding, it is our physiology that produces the end results of illness.

So the modern over-stressed human being chooses to indulge in physical exercise as a remedial activity. While previous generations who lived in simpler times got plenty of exercise daily as a matter of course, we consciously choose to exercise as a pastime, and often because of the knowledge of its health benefits. Strenuous exercise reproduces in the brain the physiological effects of violence, and provides the much-needed release to counterbalance the inflammatory provocation of stress.

---

[42] One can observe how people on a roller coaster will scream in fright during the ride, but find themselves giggling and laughing after getting off. This is a release mechanism.

Neurochemical Effects of Provocation

The study of acupuncture has shown that it relieves pain through at least two different mechanisms. One reduces the amount of inflammatory chemicals that cause it, another interferes with the nerve signals that cause the patient to perceive it. In addition to these two, there are the theories detailed in the prior chapter on acupuncture.

Although research in recent years has been focused on acupuncture, the mechanisms of action certainly apply to the other types of therapy as covered in this book. Spinal manipulation, massage, electro-therapy, etc., can interrupt nerve signals from nociceptors to the spinal cord and thence to the brain.

Although it does not penetrate the skin, Bowen Therapy movements can inhibit pressure-sensitive receptors in the skin (Merkel cells) and prevent nociceptive signals from reaching the spinal cord. Merkel cells may have a dual action on hormonal receptors as well, which is in line with the author's feeling that the major acupuncture points are neuroendocrine regulatory reflexes.

It is reasonable to assume that joint manipulation, as well as acupuncture and soft tissue manipulation like Bowen Therapy, can release naturally occurring opiate-based substances in the body. The opioid *dynorphin* is believed to lead to increased tolerance to chronic inflammatory pain[43].

Acupuncture has been found to release serotonin in the central nervous system[44]. Serotonin is well known for its ability to block descending inhibiting pathways in the brain

---

[43] Huang C, et al. *Electroacupuncture effects in a rat model of complete Freund's adjuvant-induced inflammatory pain: antinociceptive effects enhanced and tolerance development accelerated.* Neurochem Res, October 2008;33(10):2107-11.

[44] Lin JG, Chen WL. *Acupuncture analgesia: a review of its mechanisms of actions.* Am J Chin Med, 2008;36(4):635-45

that will block pain pathways in the dorsal horn, preventing pain signals from reaching the brain.

Acupuncture's ability to affect neurological pathways that stimulate the sympathetic nervous system has been seen by some as the mechanism by which it reduces pain associated with inflammation[45]. Polymodal nociceptors, one of the three types of nociceptors involved in pain perception, induce inflammatory signaling through the SNS. Various types of electro-therapy, including but not limited to electro-acupuncture, have a long track record in inhibition of just such signals. Massage has a dynamic action on sympathetic nerve stress, and must be included in any discussion about this mechanism of pain relief.

A study shows that acupuncture releases *anandamide*, a derivative of arachadonic acid, from the tissues[46]. Anandamide acts as a neurotransmitter for cannabinoid receptors that inhibit nociceptive signals.

The non-steroidal anti-inflammatory drug field has been dominated in recent years by cyclooxygenase-2 (Cox-2) inhibitors, such as ibuprofen. Acupuncture has been found to suppress Cox-2 in the spinal cord[47], as well as diminishing the potency of interleukin-1 (IL-1) and nitric oxide (NO), two pro-inflammatory chemicals. Once again, it is unreasonable to assume that only sticking needles in the skin has this effect; that is, other types of provocation (soft tissue manipulation or spinal manipulation, etc.) can produce these responses.

---

[45] Kim HW, et al. *Low-frequency electroacupuncture suppresses carrageenan-induced paw inflammation in mice via sympathetic post-ganglionic neurons, while high-frequency EA suppression is mediated by the sympathoadrenal medullary axis.* Brain Res Bull, March 28, 2008;75(5):698-705.

[46] Chen L, et al. *Endogenous anandamide and cannabinoid receptor-2 contribute to electroacupuncture analgesia in rats.* J Pain, July 2009;10(7):732-9.

[47] Lau WK, et al. *Electroacupuncture inhibits cyclooxygenase-2 up-regulation in rat spinal cord after spinal nerve ligation.* Neuroscience, Aug. 13, 2008;155(2):463-8.

The reason for pointing out the multiple documented mechanisms of action for acupuncture at this point is to illustrate that (1) there *is* more than one mechanism, and (2) there is more than one way of eliciting these mechanisms than acupuncture. *All the therapies reviewed here act mechanically, chemically, and neurologically...and possibly in other ways we have yet to understand. Uni-Syn is a way of eliciting these mechanisms more reliably and getting the most out of them.*

Regional and Referred Effects of the Provoked Points

In addition to the traditional teaching of *meridians* as the pathways of signals sent to and from the skin, in Japanese acupuncture there is the concept of Hirata's Zones, sometimes referred to as "convergent channels". These bands of tissue, delineated by acupuncturist Kurakichi Hirata, form a neural "warning system" of organic dysfunction, which is used as a diagnostic tool by palpating the different areas for tenderness, or taking into account where the patient has become spontaneously tender. Of course, these "convergent channels" are known to make that convergence at the spinal column, and Hirata was bringing traditional acupuncture a little closer to modern anatomical knowledge.

Hirata's Zones

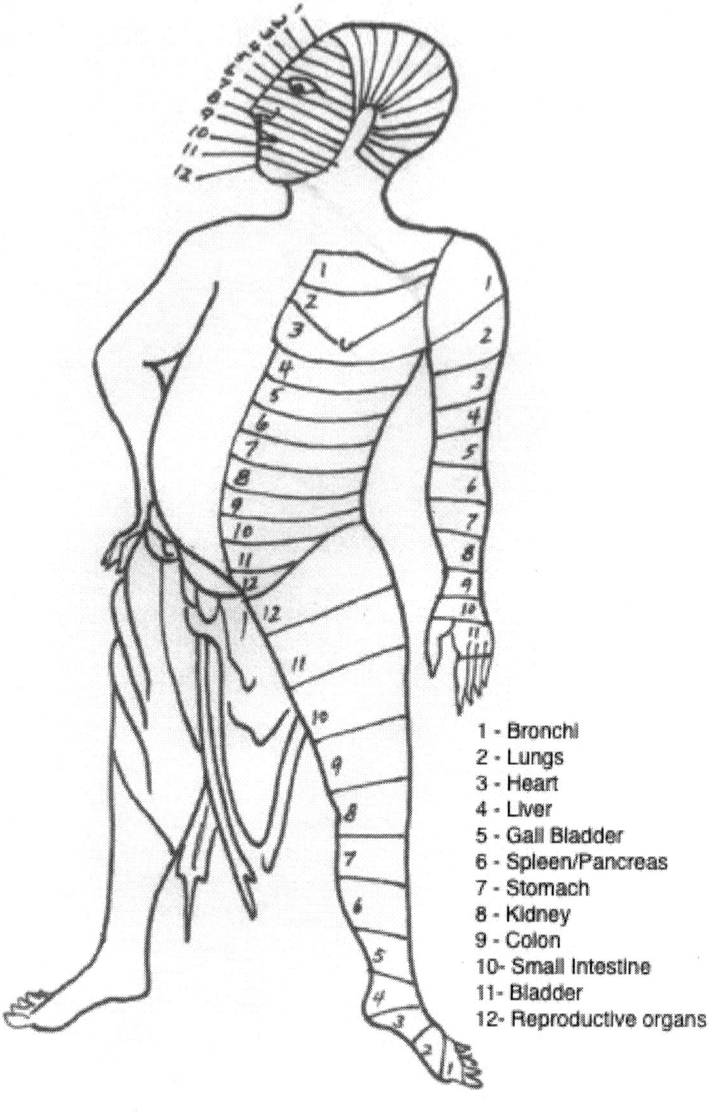

Hirata's Zones are not talked about much outside of Japanese acupuncture. Acupuncture in Japan is generally more aligned with confirmed anatomical and physiological knowledge and tends to be more science-based in its attitudes. The emphasis, therefore, is more on the predictable effects of stimulating specific points, and less on the classical Chinese explanations of how it happens, particularly the "TCM" model.

One defining difference between Eastern and Western medicine is Eastern medicine's eagerness to use empirical discoveries for practical benefit. All too often, scientific knowledge in the West increases in an area that results in no new application of that knowledge, and no new benefit as well. To illustrate, it is interesting to compare Hirata's Zones with Head's Zones.

Over a hundred years ago Sir Henry Head, an English physician, also established a neurological concept that bears his name. Head's Zones are areas of skin that "exhibit reflex hyperesthesia and hyperalgesia due to visceral disease". Head documented hundreds of cases where extra-sensitive or even painful skin coincided with organic dysfunction. He measured skin tenderness and temperature and particularly observed the pattern of rashes and pain produced by herpes zoster (shingles).

Today Head's Zones are thought to be synonymous with dermatomes, and every medical student learns about them. The phenomenon of Head's Zones is explained by the mechanism of viscerocutaneous reflexes[48]. Although every medical student is required to learn these organ-to-skin reflexes as a diagnostic tool, it is still poorly understood, even after a century. And with the emphasis on laboratory diagnosis today and the shift away from physical diagnosis, only the occasional clinician will be seen gaining information from touching the patient.

---

[48] Viscero- and somatoafferent (nociceptive) neurons are thought to meet at the lateral column of the spinal cord, but the exact location has never been determined.

Florian Beissner, Christian Henke, and Paul Unschuld, in their paper *"Forgotten Features of Head Zones and Their Relation to Diagnostically Relevant Acupuncture Points"*[49] expressed their surprise at the correlation of Head's discoveries and the much older teachings of acupuncture:

> When investigating the parallels of Western and Chinese ideas, we were astonished by the high degree of correspondence between these two systems. It is more than just historically interesting that the Chinese discovery of viscerocutaneous reflexes and their underlying systematics probably preceded the discovery in the West by more than 2000 years. Additionally one may ask, whether there is something more we can learn for today's medicine.
>
> The most important difference between Western and Chinese concepts is that in the West Head's Zones are purely used as a diagnostic tool. In all cases, the diagnosis will be checked by means of more advanced techniques. In Chinese medicine, however, Mu and Shu points are both diagnostically and therapeutically relevant. When a point is aching or when pressure on the point relieves an existing pain, this point is considered for treatment with acupuncture, moxibustion or related techniques. It is this simple idea to take a reversed action—from the skin to the viscera—for granted, which makes the Chinese concept so intriguing."

Beissner, Henke, and Unschuld point out that a striking component of Head's work that has been completely forgotten is his concept of "maximum points". Head actually

---

49 *Evidence-Based Complementary and Alternative Medicine,* Vol. 2011, Article ID 240653,http://dx.doi.org/10.1093/ecam/nen088

ascribed this discovery with having greater importance than his famous zones, yet this aspect of his work is rarely referenced.

Head found that what he called "maximum points" coincided with visceral disease. He observed that maximum points would appear, for example, where the first blisters would appear in a case of shingles, and the spread of the rash would be predictable.

He experimented with surface irritants such as mustard oil to see if any stimulation, not just digital pressure, would stimulate the maximum points and activate reflexes that would cause visceral reactions. It did.

Head's Zones

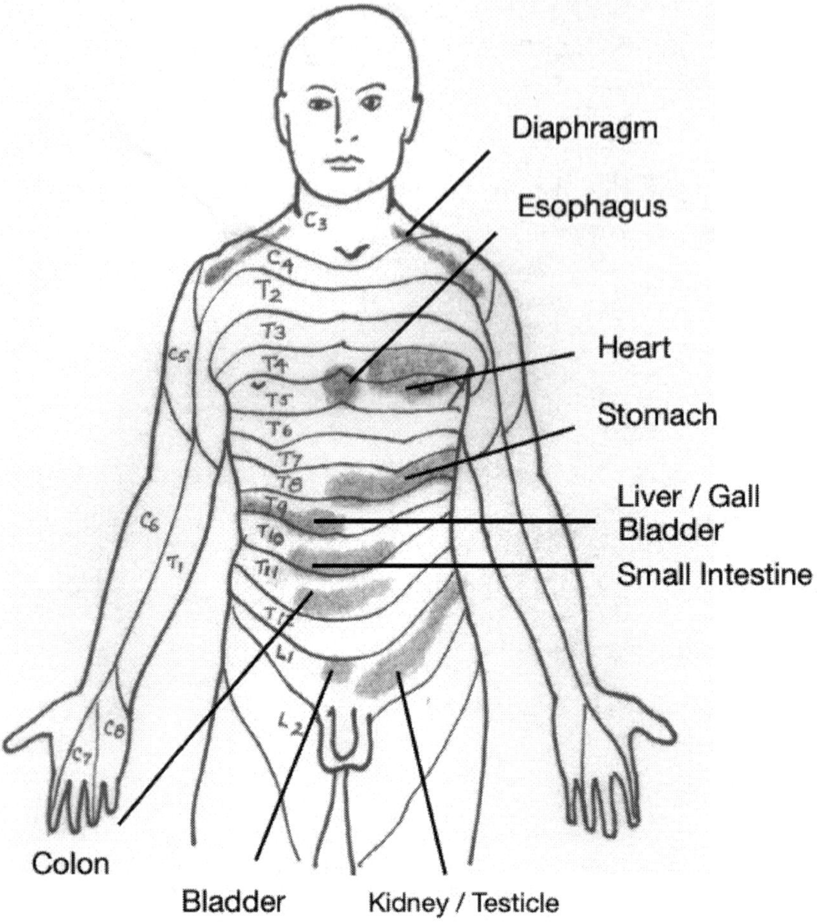
Diaphragm
Esophagus
Heart
Stomach
Liver / Gall Bladder
Small Intestine
Colon
Bladder
Kidney / Testicle

A few of Head's important statements regarding maximum points:

- "Every such area of cutaneous tenderness has one or more maximum points, the position of which is exceedingly important, for it is to the situation of these maxima that the patient refers his pain"[50].
- "There is great cutaneous tenderness...Yet firm deep pressure relieves, rather than aggravates, his pain"[51].
- "Thus, mustard leaves applied to the maximum spots of the affected areas of the chest or back...will remove the nausea and vomiting in this mild and purely reflex type of gastric disturbance"[52].

Head could have been talking about acu-pressure, Shiatsu, or Neuromuscular Therapy for all the similarity of his observation that deep pressure relieved pain in areas of surface tenderness.

Using a superficial irritant, such as mustard oil, to elicit internal reactions proves that a mechanical force is not necessary to activate reflexes. The important thing is to have the correct neurological pathway to the target organ or structure.

As Beissner, Henke, and Unschuld stress in their discussion of Head's work, conventional Western medicine can use Head's Zones for diagnostic purposes, but Asian medicine also uses them for therapeutic purposes, sending a signal back to the spine and then to the dysfunctional organ.

---

50 [H. Head, "On disturbances of sensation with especial reference to the pain of visceral disease," *Brain*, vol. 16, p. 6]

51 *Ibid*, p. 71

52 *Ibid*, p.261

Spinal + Distal Provocation

An example of a combination of regional and distant sites of provocation can be seen in the matter of voiding disorders. The mainstream medical journal *Urology* published a study in 2008[53] showing that electro-acupuncture was effective in relieving male voiding dysfunction by using just three sets of points: UB-32, UB-33, and GB-30 (which we will later see as being part of a standard Uni-Syn protocol). These points are all located in the sacral region.

Sacral electrical stimulation, both by implanted electrodes and also surface electrodes, has been shown to be effective for urinary incontinence and frequent urination in other trials. The areas stimulated were the second through fourth sacral foramina, coincidentally where the same acupuncture points related to the urinary bladder reside. The researchers concluded that the electromagnetic fields generated by the stimulation affects the cauda equina and the cutaneous nerve of the surface of the sacrum, and created responses from the primary somatosensory cortex[54].

But another reliable way to address this disorder is by use of a distal point that acts as a "remote control" button for the genitourinary organs, which acupuncturists all know as Spleen-Pancreas point #6. Once again, the unity of acupuncture and conventionally-understood neurological effects can be seen.

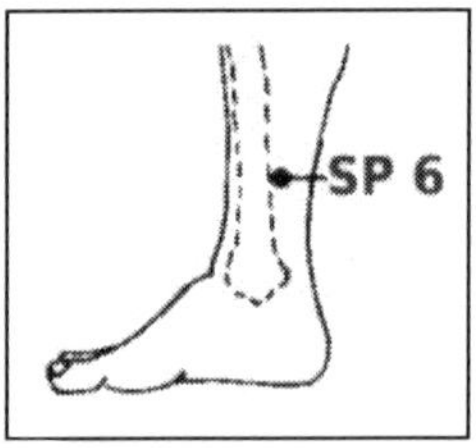

Electrical stimulation of the posterior tibial nerve has also been found effective in bladder disorders[55]. It affects the lower pelvic contents by way of brain perception of the signal thus created, and the brain sends a return signal to inhibit

---

53 Lee, S., Lee, B.; *Eletcroacupuncture Relieves Pain In Men With Chronic Prostatitis/ Chronic Pelvic Pain Syndrome: Three-Arm Randomized Trial*; Urology 2008, 10/047

54 *Neurosci Lett,* 2008 Jan 24;431(1):77-80

55 *Posterior Tibial Nerve Electrical Stimulation*, Dialogues in Ped Urol, June 2011:5-6

spasm (as Tom Bowen so simply and eloquently expressed it in his Bowen Therapy). The posterior tibial nerve is a mixed peripheral sensory-motor nerve. Originating from the spinal roots of L4-S3, it affects sensory and also motor control of the pelvic floor, bladder and bladder sphincter, and also the anal sphincter as well. Stimulation of this nerve creates central inhibition of pre-ganglionic motor neurons in the bladder through a spinal cord route.

The traditional acupuncturist will prefer to attribute these effects to a meridian mechanism, although the neurological underpinnings are beyond question. Western clinical researchers, on the other hand, studiously avoid any mention of acupuncture in their papers. Yet the illustration of the method just discussed clearly showed *an acupuncture needle being used* in a standard electroacupuncture protocol when it was published. Sadly, it is still injudicious for medical doctors to give credence to acupuncture. But it is also often injudicious for acupuncturists to admit to neurological mechanisms in what have been traditionally seen as "energy effects".

Whichever "turf" one chooses to defend, it is clear that the simply stated but profound mechanism explained by Tom Bowen is there: A signal goes from the skin and fascia to the brain, it overrides the dysfunctional signals going to the brain, and the brain sends a healing signal back down to the area.

What more do we need to understand?

Summation

- What the author calls the "venting points", in addition to meeting the criteria for classification as trigger points, represents a localized inflammatory response as well as a focus for the body to attempt to discharge metabolic wastes.
- These points need to be stimulated to mobilize what classical acupuncturists would call "stagnant energy" or "excess *qi*".
- Stimulation should cause some sensation in order to activate the *deqi* effect (sensation of stimulation). Creating *deqi* causes a strong sensation that in turn causes a "reawakening" of sorts in the brain.
- Areas in the brain often have lowered activity due to chronic pain, and establish a "numbing" effect. This is dispersed under treatment as the "acupuncture effect" reactivates those brain regions.
- Provocation in Uni-Syn can be accomplished with various means:
    - Manual pressure (Collins technic, NMT, Bowen, Shiatsu, etc.)
    - T-bar or other manual tool
    - Injection of medicinal substances (as in Neural Therapy)
    - Acupuncture needle
    - *Teishin* (spring-loaded non-invasive "needle")
    - Activator-type spring-loaded tool
    - Mechanical vibrator with a protruding head
    - Electrical stimulation (Piezo, unipolar, bipolar, etc.)

While effective stimulation of points on the skin to cause distant effects can certainly be achieved with non-sensory means, such as lasers, the author recommends those sensation-causing methods outlined above.

The acceptance of the *deqi* sensation is essential not simply because of its neurochemical effects but for its psychological effects as well. People who are consciously or unconsciously resistant to change will remain locked in chronic disease patterns. And because the typical patient has been to multiple therapists, there is often denial of the likelihood of healing. Psychologically, a strong sensation during treatment must be created for these people, to impart a sense of something powerful happening and to overcome the denial of ability of the therapy to change the condition[56].

Everyone must make a breakthrough in order to heal, overcoming resistance to change, and being willing to relinquish the secondary benefits the disease gives him (in the form of sympathy, alleviation of responsibility, etc.).

---

[56] One time, when I was lamenting that an intervention had not worked, an obstinate patient told me, "Ha! My disease is stronger than your treatment!" It was more important for this patient to have some kind of power than to be free of her problems.

13

THE LAWS OF POLARITY

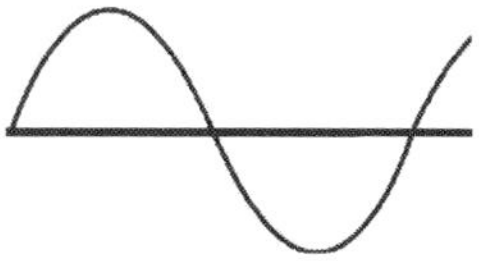

We began this book with a discussion of electrical principles, because our world is in many ways an electrical one. The surface of the earth itself is negatively charged while the ionosphere is positively charged. This leaves an eighty kilometer space between them that is an electrostatic field; it is a capacitor, in electrical terms. It stores an electric charge. The world we move in and the air we fly in is charged at 200 volts per meter. We live in a virtual battery created by opposing polarities.

It is fascinating that the human body reflects this situation all the way down to the cellular level. But before we reach the microscopic level, let us first consider the principle of Polarity as it relates to something we can actually see.

The velocity of blood—that is, the speed at which it passes a certain point—changes with the location in the body. In the aorta the velocity is high during systole and almost nil during diastole. Yet, in the smaller arteries, the velocity is less during systole and great during diastole. The “yin-yang” relationship of these phenomena is obvious. When there is fullness, there is corresponding emptiness, and vice-versa. *No less an important apparatus than the heart maintains this polarity principle at all times.*

Biochemical Polarity

At the cellular level, polarity is at work constantly. All types of cells rely on electrical charges to initiate the energy that runs cellular functions. Electrolytes are minerals that are suspended in a colloidal solution, which is capable of producing electrical charges within (intracellular[57]) and between the cells (extracellular[58]). It could be said that this dynamic corresponds to what the ancient Chinese referred to as *qi* flow.

Electrolytes conduct electrical impulses as their minerals dissociate into polarized ions. This process is connected to many processes—pH balance in the fluids; adrenal gland mineral-corticoid function; digestion and assimilation of nutrients—and as such, electrolyte solutions have an impact on every tissue and function of the body. When electrolytes are imbalanced there is haphazard conductivity, affecting electrical flow through the cells.

Bodily fluids are negatively-charged colloidal solutions. Since similarly-charged particles repel each other, there is a normal system of checks to maintain a balance between attraction and repulsion of particles.

Many common diseases have their source in an electrolyte imbalance—either excess or deficiency. The polarity of these conditions and their underlying mineral states can be seen in the following chart.

---

[57] Blood cells, parenchymal cells of organs, vascular endothelial cells.

[58] Blood plasma, lymphatic fluid, interstitial fluid

HIGH (electrolyte stress)	LOW (electrolyte insufficiency)
Excess concentrations of electrolytes	Low concentrations of electrolytes
Excess electrical conductivity	Low electrical conductivity
Hypertension	Hypotension
Nervous tension	Nervous exhaustion
Blood agglutination	Anemia
Platelet aggregation	Low platelets
High plasma volume	Low plasma volume
Adrenal stress	Adrenal fatigue
Kidney stress	Kidney fatigue
Cardiac stress	Cardiac fatigue
Low minerals from salt aggregation	Low minerals from poor retention
Tendency toward heated states	Tendency toward cold states
"Excess" conditions (i.e., migraines)	"Deficiency" conditions (i.e., dull headaches)

While we can observe polarity effects in typical physiological processes, and in disease states, the methods for correcting them also have their polar attributes. Consider these manifestations of polarity changes in various therapies:

- Illnesses are observed to change from acute (+) to chronic (-).
- Illnesses are observed to progress from inflammatory (+) to degenerative (-).
- Traditional Oriental medicine describes a change in pathology over time, from increased *yang* (+) to decreased *yang* and increased *yin* (-).
- Measuring the acupuncture points with methods such as electrodermal screening (EDS) shows high conductivity (+) of related points in inflammatory or acute conditions, progressing to falling values on the gauge ("indicator drop") when the condition has progressed to a degenerative one (-).
- Chiropractic doctors using a Nervoscope to measure spinal segments will see evidence of heat (+) at the site of a bulging disk, but the temperature becomes subnormal (-) when that disk thins after time, or after rupturing.
- Homeopathic doctors apply a medicine that in normal strength would *cause* the combination of symptoms the patient is experiencing, and thus "trick" the system into anticipating a dramatic increase in the symptoms. Because of the predictable polarizing reaction of the body, symptoms then move from their peak toward the opposite pole. "Like poles repel, unlike poles attract."
- Allopathic doctors prescribe a medicine that opposes the symptoms produced by the body, forcing them to move in the opposite direction. The polarizing reaction of the body is to increase its efforts in the original direction; hence, stronger doses of the medicine are needed over time ("oral tolerance").

Polarity in the Nervous System

At the level of the nervous system, polarity principles are at work all the time. Nerves transmit their signals by means of depolarization, which creates something known as *action potential.* The cell membrane is said to be polarized because the fluid inside it has a negative electrical charge while the outside is positively charged. When the ions of potassium and sodium are balanced, the cell is said to be resting. Then a buildup of positively charged potassium in the nerve cell escapes from the cell toward negatively-charged sodium outside the cell, which floods into the cell. Because the cell membrane is semipermeable, these elements can travel in both directions through ion channels that are activated by ATP. This reversal of the polarity—suddenly negative inside and positive outside—creates the voltage (about +30 mV) that is the nerve impulse. Then the nerve cell returns to what is called *resting potential* and re-polarization with the inside positively charged and the outside negative. It is an alternating process, creating an on/off electrical impulse. Remember the illustration of piezoelectricity? This is an important point to consider, as we shall see shortly in our discussion of the Law of Periodicity.

The Neurolemma

The *neurolemma* (also known as neurilemma or "sheath of Schwann") is the outermost layer surrounding the axon of a neuron. If the nerve is the electric cable of the human body, the neurolemma is the insulation covering it. It is made of a nucleated cytoplasmic layer of what are called Schwann cells, and is the outermost layer of nerve fibers in the peripheral nervous system. In anatomy and physiology classes, it is taught that its function is simply to insulate a nerve from its neighboring nerve, to isolate the transmission of nerve impulses so that they are not jumbled with other messages from the brain (as in the case of neurological diseases like Multiple Sclerosis and ALS, where the insulation is lost off the nerves).

But the research of Robert O. Becker, MD (mentioned previously) showed that the neurolemma has another vital function: that of carrying electrically transmitted information. His work on the healing process of bone fractures revealed that a measurable direct current flows along the neurolemma, and that this DC current commands the healing process and directs RNA coding to the affected tissues, near and far. This is in contrast to the digital signal traveling through the nerves themselves—nerve impulses are simply on or off. A DC signal makes possible more complex transmission of information.

The work of Becker shows that the ancient concept of blockages along the acupuncture meridians is revealing something valid, something that can be measured and explained in light of present-day anatomical knowledge (which was always the stumbling block for Western physicians regarding acupuncture). Resistance can build up at various spots (sites of trauma, etc.) and partially block the transmission of this analog signal that directs the healing response.

Becker's work in regenerating limbs that have been excised from salamanders[59] showed significant polarity characteristics. Becker's hypothesis is that trauma (including surgical trauma) sets up a "current of injury" that creates a heightened positive polarity voltage in the tissues that gradually falls into a negative polarity, which marks the healing response. When the healing is completed, the polarity is again neutral. This was observed in his work healing spinal cord injury in salamanders and goldfish. Becker observed that the longer the positive polarity current was present, the less likely spinal regeneration was to occur.

It is the contention of this work that Uni-Syn, and in fact *all* therapies when applied judiciously, do nothing more than provoke this same response. When the healing process is at a standstill or terminates prematurely, a therapy that jogs

---

[59] Detailed in *The Body Electric,* by Becker and Selden; William Morrow Pub., 1998.

that response to the current of injury will restore the natural reversing of that injury. In other words, sometimes the current of injury continues unabated in the positive polarity range, as exemplified by chronic inflammation, for example. A good therapy mimics the catalytic action that occurs when

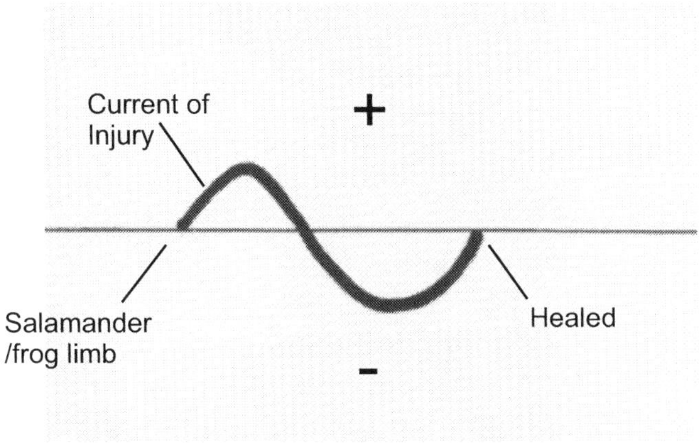

the nervous system begins to reverse the polarity at the site of injury. It is the small "trauma" that causes the brain to once again recognize that something needs attention, in the same way that a highly diluted homeopathic medicine excites the attention of the nervous system because it carries a hint of a toxic substance. For this reason, we prefer to use a provocation method in Uni-Syn that causes some sensation; a micro-trauma. Or, as acupuncturists put it, the *de qi* effect.

Since we know that emotionally, people not only respond to injury but also the *threat* of injury, it follows that the body-mind system can do likewise ("If you press on me any harder, I might be injured!"). Remedial efforts jog the healing response because their stimulation causes the brain to interpret them as new insults that must be healed.

It is difficult to have a satisfying blend of humanistic concepts and hard science, and this book may be challenging for some in both camps. But Becker's goldfish and salamanders who grew back their parts are objective evidence that these concepts are not simply wishful theorizing.

When viewing the venerable yin-yang symbol of acupuncture, or the heady illustrations of Polarity Therapy[60] (with its correspondences of elements and symbols and body parts), a metaphysical atmosphere is created that is immediately viewed with suspicion by the scientifically-trained mind. Yet, the same principles and actions are seen every day in the cold, dispassionate study of physiology. The same events, when seen under a microscope, lose their global implications—observing a nerve cell at work does not *seem* to tell you anything about how to dose a medicine, how to twirl an inserted needle, how to pace a bodywork session, how much time to allow between treatments, etc.

The problem to date is that those with a mastery of the scientific underpinnings of health care have such a narrow focus that they do not see the "big picture", and those who focus exclusively on the "big picture" often become scattered and overly-theoretical. Both limit their effectiveness as providers.

Polarity of Light and Color

The perception of a particular color depends on a predominance of frequencies in a given part of the spectrum being present in the light being viewed. When enough of that color has been absorbed by the eye, closing the eye will produce an interesting phenomenon: the opposite color will appear. For example, if blue light has been viewed, an orange color will be seen with the eyes closed.

Chromotherapy, a special type of light therapy utilizing colored light, was extensively researched and developed in the last century. The most well-known developer of this method was Dinshah. Having used the Dinshah system of chromotherapy clinically for many years, I came to realize that the typical indications for a particular color to be

---

[60] A conceptual therapy originated by Randolph Stone, DC, ND, DO, derived from Chiropractic, Acupuncture, Yoga, and Ayurveda, and focusing on the flow of "life energies" in the body.

applied to a given case were effective in an acute condition, but less effective in a chronic one. When I tried using the opposite color for these cases I found that, far from exacerbating the condition, it helped resolve it more surely. As an example, acute inflammation would be typically treated with blue light. But chronic inflammation responded better to red light, which theoretically should have worsened it. I came to realize that acute conditions needed to be treated, so to speak, in an antipathic way while chronic conditions should be treated in a homeopathic way. In other words, "the hair of the dog that bit you". Rubor (redness) being a characteristic of inflammation, red light created a rebound response in the tissues and created a resolution of the condition.

Meteorological Polarity

Large prairie fires on the Midwestern plains have always been observed to cause strong rains. This is an example of homeopathicity (the underlying principle of homeopathic medicine), as well as polarity and *periodicity* (discussed in the next chapter).

How is it homeopathic? The prolonged heat and dryness on the ground, matched with the heat and dryness in the atmosphere, results in an opposing reaction: rain. Thus it is at the same time an illustration of polarity and periodicity, where the cycle of heat and dryness gives way to cooler temperatures and humidity.

To diverge for a moment: A good illustration of how the Law of Polarity is a universal one can be seen in the decidedly non-physical realm of economics. The principle of "supply and demand" plays out this theme constantly. For example, as prices rise, real estate investors build more houses. When the supply floods the market, it drives the prices down again.

"Opposites Attract"

This universal observation is expressed in proverb form in almost every culture. If one looks beyond the simple generalization, one will see that this truism reflects the Law of Polarity. In this way, one will also see that the Uni-Syn principles have a marked application toward understanding and affecting psychosocial states. Our interactions with others can be analyzed and understood by viewing them within the framework of the principles described here.

One example will suffice for now. Everyone has encountered those dispassionate characters who are considered "cool". Unflappable, their appeal to others lies in their detachment. Fictional characters like James Bond and real-life personalities like Dean Martin are good illustrations. The rest of us wish that we too were as unaffected by stress, and difficult circumstances. We wish that we kept our composure as well as these gentlemen, but unfortunately most of us experience varying degrees of passion that cause us to explode in a rage, or laugh at our own jokes, or be nervous or impatient, etc.

Now it is also well observed that these "cool" characters are attractive to those who are unlike them. It is also well known that the more that attractive people of either sex play "hard to get", the more they are pursued by their admirers. I would propose that this is nothing more than an expression of the Law of Polarity (also expressed in the folk wisdom that "opposites attract").

Like poles repel and unlike poles attract.

If one imagines the now-familiar median line dividing the positive and negative phases of polarity, one could picture the dispassionate Dean Martin as creating a greater deviation from the mean in the negative phase than normal. If passion and detachment in perfect balance represent a mild sine wave with no great rise or fall (Fig. 1), a large degree of unemotional calm could be seen as a negative phase wave (Fig. 2). In the world of chemistry, when there is a solution of greater gravity on one side of a permeable membrane, the increased osmotic pressure causes a migration of fluid through the membrane to the other side. In this illustration, the large absence of passion, if we can call it that, represents a negative pressure or vacuum that draws its opposite toward it, from the opposite side of the dividing line (Fig. 3).

Fig. 1

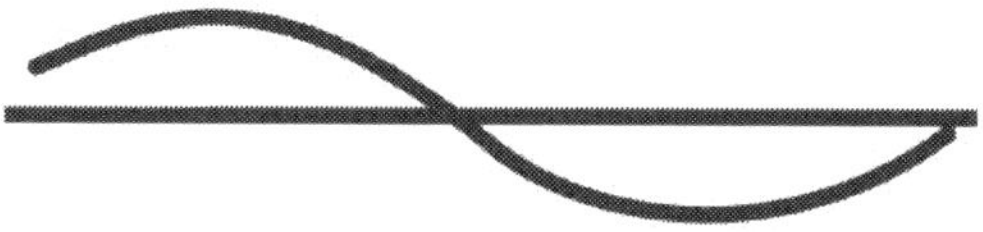

Passion balanced
with detachment

Fig. 2

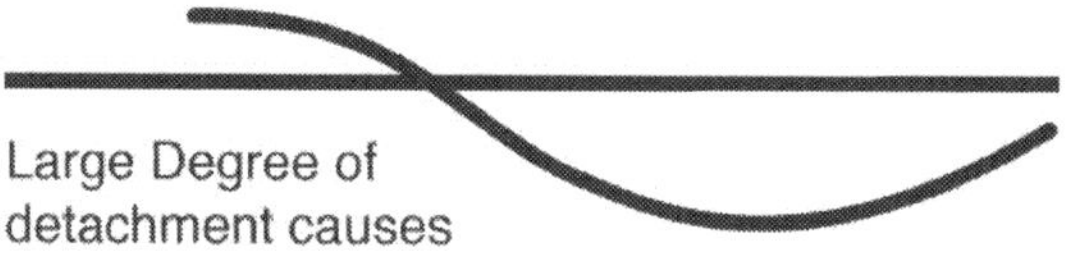

Large Degree of
detachment causes
vacuum effect...

Fig. 3

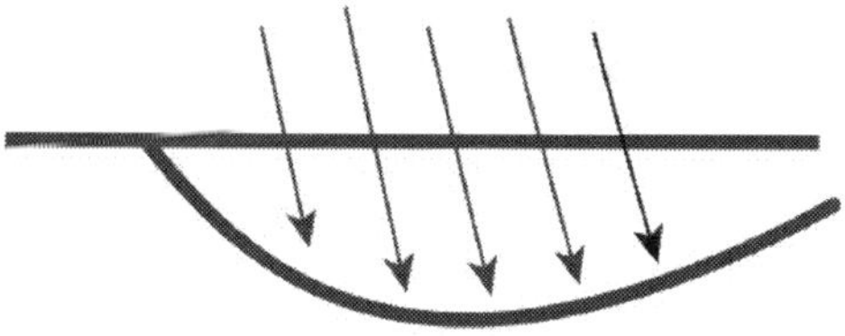

... that causes movement toward
the pole with the greater amplitude,
like osmosis

Of course, this is purely symbolic and for illustrative purposes only. I am not suggesting that any kind of measurable energy shift occurs in the example of personalities given. However, it may just be that we can understand and predict human behavior much better if we take the trouble to map out interactions according to the known laws discussed here. There may be no detectable mechanism for it, but who is to say that psychosocial actions and reactions could not mirror those of the electrical and chemical worlds? This is all about *patterns*, and the observation of reliable patterns leads to more predictable outcomes.

Adaptation Response

Hippocrates, the father of medicine, wrote that the disease process was composed of both *pathos* (suffering) and *ponos* (toil). The innate response to the suffering is the effort to restore balance and normal functioning. An intact homeostatic mechanism in the body leads to corrections (and therefore health), while a maladaptive response leads to chronic illness as the body first resists the pattern, then becomes exhausted by it.

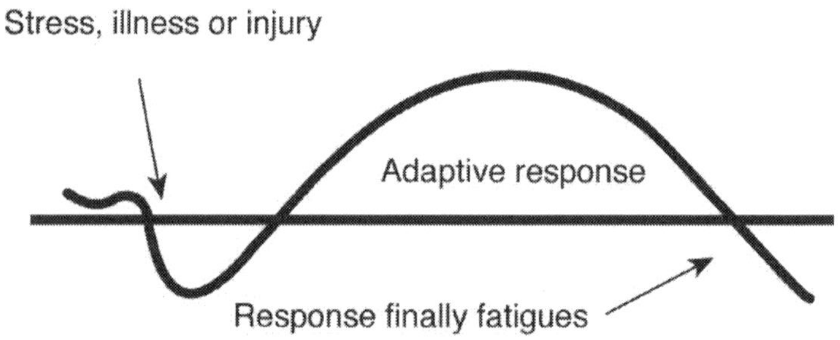

While this physiological fact is recognized by all schools of medicine, its polarity characteristics are invisible until displayed in this manner; the old familiar sine wave appears when it is illustrated this way. Once adaptive response, and in particular a maladaptive response, is recognized as a polarity phenomenon, it is easier to predict changes in the patient's condition and easier to apply the correct therapy at the proper time.

Polarity expresses itself in many of the rhythms of nature. If we view one 24-hour period, the circadian rhythm of the day reveals the hallowed *yin-yang* or sine wave, with its alternating polarities:

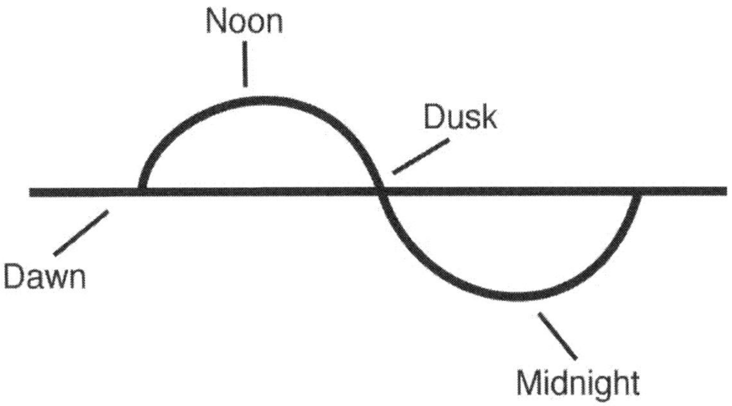

And when viewed from a year's perspective, the same applies to seasons:

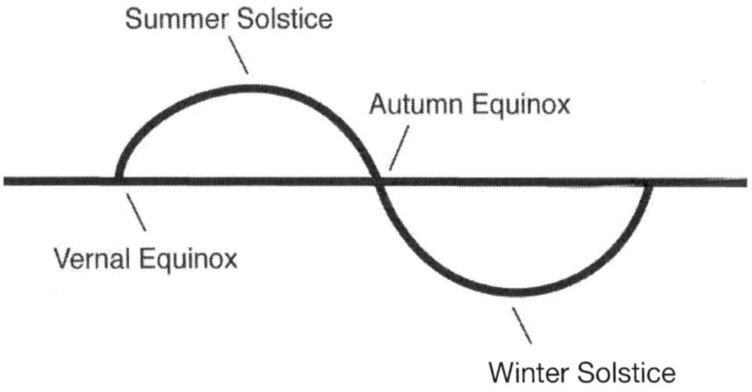

Another way to visualize it provides a more powerful image with which to understand the predictable evolution of the seasons:

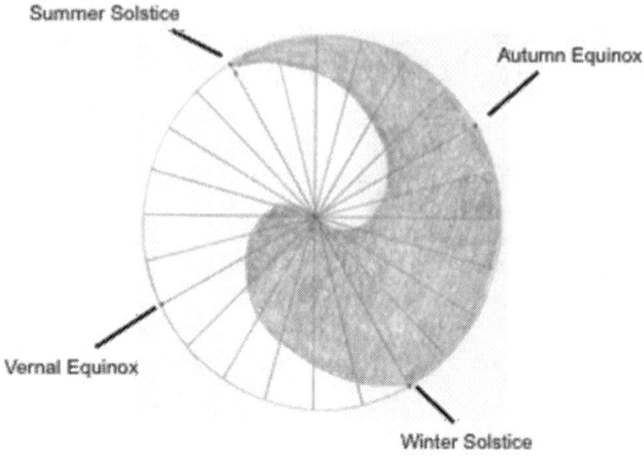

This type of illustration provides a good segue into the next related principle, *Periodicity*.

14

THE LAWS OF PERIODICITY

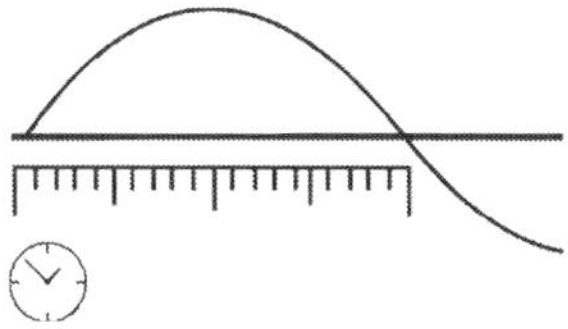

The life spans of domestic animals are fairly predictable and have not changed over time: 15-20 years for cats, 10-20 years for dogs, 30-50 years for horses, etc. Why do elephants live 60-70 years? Simply because they are bigger and can hold more years? Guinea pigs live a short time while a turtle the same size as the Guinea pig lives a long time. The life span of an animal seems to be something that is pre-programmed, or at least follows certain predictable patterns.

While life expectancy for humans has increased in the U.S. in the past 100 years, what has not changed is the *mortality-doubling time.* This is the length of time it takes for the likelihood of death to double. At age 45, a person has twice the risk of dying as that same person did at age 37 or 38. In another 7-8 years, it doubles again. In fact, insurance company actuary tables track this bit of information, and the policy premium rates increase accordingly at the same time intervals. Obviously, the insurance industry banks on reliable predictors, and this seems to be one.

What is fascinating is that this timing appears to be unchanged even by external factors. A study of Australian prisoners in Japanese concentration camps during World War II showed that the mortality-doubling time there was still the same, even though the death rate was *ten times higher* than outside the camps.[61]

Even though we are living longer, aging is not slowing down, despite claims of "anti-aging" products. Olympic athletes, for example, are still people in their twenties. *If aging was proportionate to life span, they would now be in their forties.*

If the rate at which we age remains fixed, even if we are able to squeeze out a few more years than we were able to a century ago, then what other cycles are at work of which we may be unaware?

It is the author's conviction that such natural cycles increase or decrease (depending on how they are utilized) the likelihood of therapies being successful, as we shall see.

Cycles of Action, Cycles of Rest

It is well known that weight lifting must be performed on alternate days at most for continuous progress in muscle-building. Without rest periods between sessions, the muscle fatigue will prevent steady growth. A period of rebuilding is necessary to achieve the objective.

Morris Krok, one of the first Western writers on the subject of yoga, pointed out in the 1940s that Hatha Yoga postures

> ...consist of a period of tension which is followed by a period of relaxation. This arrangement is in accordance with the physiological activities of the human body where a resting interval always follows a period of exertion or contraction.[62]

This is an illustration of the Law of Polarity at the same time; the passive *yin* must counterbalance the active *yang*. But it

[61] *J Gerontol* 48; 3:14-20

[62] Krok, *Hatha Yoga —the Vibrant Science of Life*, 1975

also presents in very clear terms the Law of Periodicity. **The action that appears to be the purpose of the activity—lifting weights, holding a yoga pose, massaging a tender spot, stimulating an acupuncture point, taking a medicine, manipulating a joint, etc.—is nothing without its invisible counterbalancing-and-developing rest period.**

One can see from this graph that when correctly done, exercise produces gains in strength, endurance, agility, etc., when periodicity is respected. As exercise is applied, there is fatigue, soreness, and other responses to the work. If given a proper recovery time, more work can be done than previously as the body adapts to, and actually becomes capable of, a higher intensity of work.[63] Over time and repetition, the body gains new ability. Challenging exercise plus rest periods creates consistent progress. On the other hand, exercise that is too easy causes loss of progress after a time.

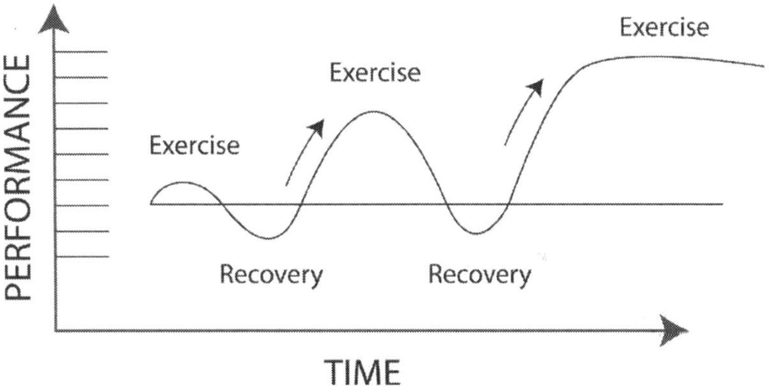

Furthermore, the Law of Periodicity as it applies to exercise has great import for therapies as well. Progress in therapy exactly follows the principles of progress in exercise performance. Gains are best made by the timing of the sessions.

---

63 Recovery or rest periods, of course, must be adjusted to the work done. Intense exercise requires a longer recovery time than light exercise. If not observed, the body will not make consistent progress and can actually stagnate. Those who violate this rule can be heard to say "I keep working out but I'm getting weaker."

Most practitioners depend on a cumulative effect from repeatedly treating their patients. If they are not inadvertently using appropriate rest periods, they are simply breaking down the body's ability to produce symptoms. Judicial application of a therapy, including the rest periods, will produce actual healing.

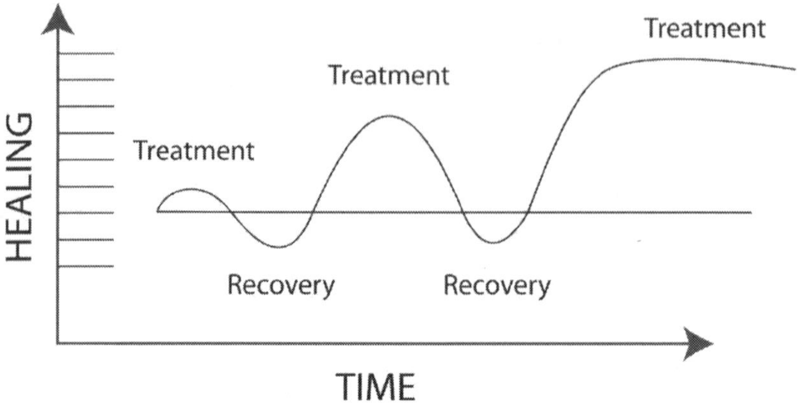

In animal training, there is a principle called "soaking" that is considered essential. When teaching an animal new behavior, a significant pause is always observed after practice drills in the new performance. This allows the new information to "soak in"—thus the term "soaking". It is based on long observation and is the key to success. Animal brains do not radically differ from human brains in this regard.

When I first encountered Bowen Therapy, the most distinctive aspect of it was the pause between segments of the applied movements. When it was explained that the pause allows the brain to process the stimulation in order to direct the healing reaction, I was fascinated. The implications for other therapies that I had already studied began suggesting themselves almost immediately.

It is interesting to note that when a horse is trained in a new conduct and the lesson "soaks in", the animal demonstrates predictable behavior. The horse will begin chewing motions, licking its lips and sticking its tongue out. The visually bizarre behavior could easily be mistaken for illness. In the same way, a human undergoing treatment for a health problem correctly—i.e., therapy followed by appropriate rest periods—will often temporarily present a worsening of symptoms, or symptoms of a new problem. The "healing crisis", as it is traditionally called by naturopaths, is likely a confirmative sign of the treatment "soaking in". Chiropractors will call it a "re-tracing" of the pattern of illness back to its source. Homeopaths say that "an aggravation is followed by amelioration", illustrating both the arousal of the healing response and the Law of Polarity at the same time (as the amplitude of the symptoms diminishes, it enters a new phase as it crosses the median in the sine wave illustration).

Chiropractors were at one time very aware of the cycles of action and rest. By the time Chiropractic had experienced its greatest period of unabated growth and settled into a popular niche relative to conventional medicine, practitioners had developed some distinct features of clinical practice. While the technics they applied to the spine sometimes varied depending on the school, chiropractors of all stripes employed a method to get better results in their offices; a method that took into account the principle of Periodicity. Chiropractic offices in the 1950s often devoted a significant amount of space to "resting rooms". In what seems to be a nearly forgotten piece of wisdom today, these doctors insisted that patients rest on cots in a relaxing atmosphere after having their spines adjusted.

The action that appears to be the purpose of the activity—lifting weights, holding a yoga pose, massaging a tender spot, stimulating an acupuncture point, taking a medicine, manipulating a joint, etc.—is nothing without its invisible counterbalancing-and-developing rest period.

In the same way that today's Bowen Therapy practitioners pause for a few minutes after a segment of maneuvers in order to allow the proper engagement of the central nervous system, chiropractors of yesteryear were using the same principle. Why this has slipped from memory in the profession since those days is pure conjecture.

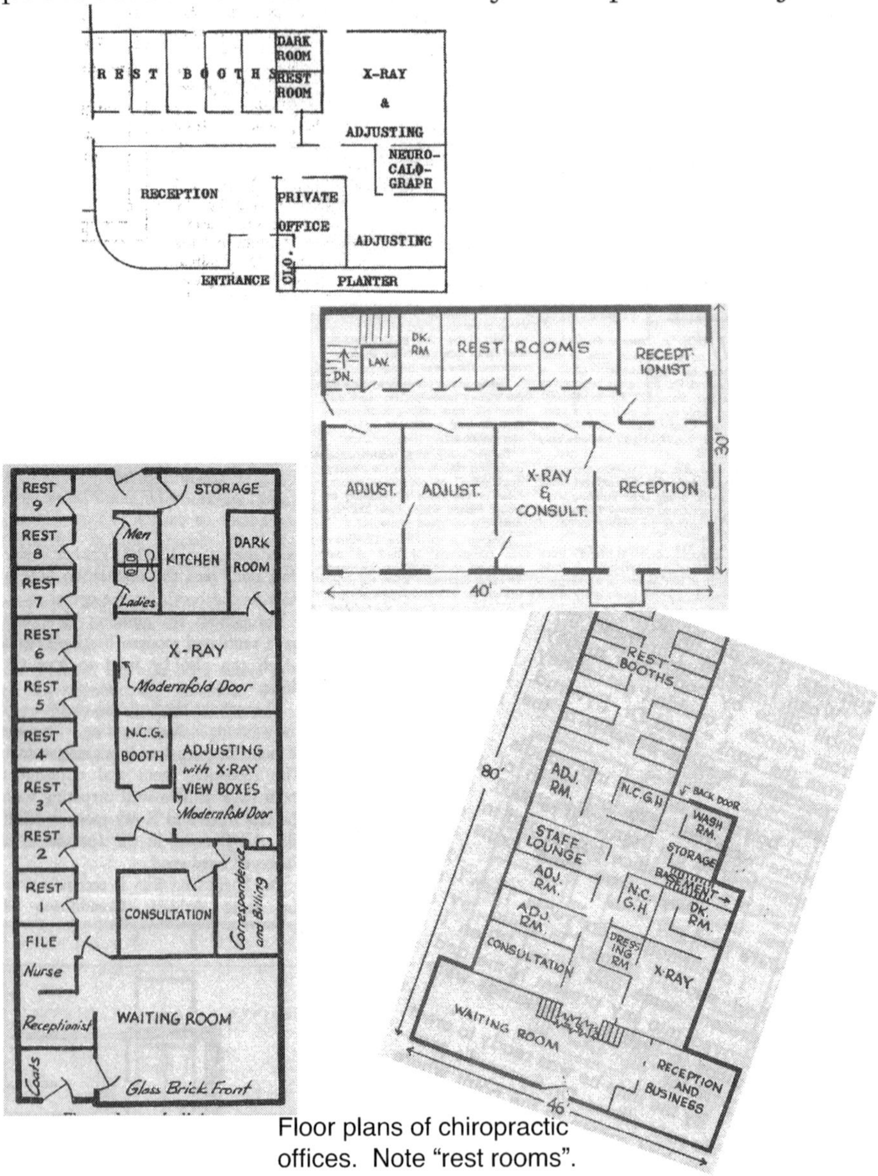

Floor plans of chiropractic offices. Note "rest rooms".

Cycles of action and cycles of rest also have a rhythm in the cyclical swing in polarity, where one length of time represents a swell of activity, and another represents a drop. In dealing with this observation, a number comes to light repeatedly, and we are referring to this as the Septimal Law.

Since ancient times, we have divided the week into seven days. This is not arbitrary or based on the Biblical account of the creation of the world in six days followed by a day of rest; it is an attempt to organize time based on the reliable observation that the moon goes through a complete cycle in twenty-eight days. Every seven days, the moon can be seen to have a predictable shape, from full to half to crescent to invisible.

Lightning strikes the earth from 2,000 to 4,000 times a day on average. They stimulate long-wave radio waves that reside in the ionosphere and the electrical energy from the lightning focuses them into low-frequency standing waves. These low-frequency waves, spread throughout the atmosphere, are known as *Schumann waves*. Toomey and Polk[64] reported that the common frequencies of these waves have been observed to be 7.8, 14.1, 20.3, and 26.4 Hz, with 14.1 Hz the most commonly found in most of the United States. One will recognize a spacing of roughly seven between these frequencies; not exact, but in the range to suggest some kind of order. It could just as easily have been a blast of random frequencies, but it was not. There is the influence of seven. The higher frequencies can be seen to be harmonics (to a degree) of the predominant 7.8 Hz frequency known as the "Schumann resonance".

In the higher ranges of the electromagnetic spectrum, we have the various wave lengths of light to consider. There, too, we find the influence of the number Seven.

---

[64] Toomey, J., Polk, C.; *Bedford*, Air Force Cambridge Research Lab, 1970

When light passes through a fluid, its beam is refracted; it is split into seven rays, giving us the colors of the rainbow and the classic mnemonic ROYGBIV (red, orange, yellow, green, blue, indigo, violet). These colors, and the half points in between (scarlet, lemon, turquoise, purple, and magenta), are used in chromotherapy, a system of light therapy using the visible parts of the light spectrum. Why does light refract into seven main colors? It simply does, and physical science takes advantage of it for spectroscopy and other uses, but does not seek to explain *why* there are seven rays.

Since the spectroscope shows us that each element emanates specific frequencies of light and can be identified by its "signature", it is a not entirely unreasonable conclusion that illness produces changes in the frequencies of light given off by the affected tissues. Chromotherapy therefore supplies the tissues with the missing frequencies of light as represented by their colors. It is known that orange light, for example, is stimulating to the thyroid gland while indigo has a depressant action on the same gland. Chromotherapy is yet another field that has a hidden "seven".

John Zimmerman of the University of Colorado did experiments to measure the electromagnetic fields of various parts of the brain to monitor the rest of the body. It was found that when a trained touch healer attempts to heal a person, there are distinct changes in those fields. Signals of up to several hundred times greater amplitude were observed when the healer was applying his method. Zimmerman observed biofields produced by healer's hands, and measured them as pulsed signals with variable frequency range, with most of the activity being in the 7 to 8 Hz range.

Henry Lindlahr, MD, who was considered one of the greatest names in natural medicine in his day, often made reference to the "Rule of Seven", discussing it in his magnum opus, *Nature Cure*. Lindlahr observed cycles that applied to disease and healing, and was the ancestor of the modern scientific naturopathic doctor.

Decades later, Victor Earl Irons (the author's ancestor) lectured about the same Rule of Seven. Among the first to use and manufacture colloidal bentonite and psyllium seed husks for detoxification purposes, Uncle Earl, as he was known in our family, was also one of the founders of the National Health Federation, and a nationally known health authority. He pointed out frequently that Nature uses units of seven in varied ways:

- The moon completes its cycle from full to new moon in 28 days
- A woman's menstrual cycle is typically 28 days
- Her baby's gestation period is typically 280 days
- Chicken eggs hatch in 21 days
- Most duck eggs hatch in 35 days

Uncle Earl taught that the body healed in cycles of seven, also: Seven days needed to cleanse the bloodstream, seven weeks to cleanse the lymphatic system, seven months to cleanse the endocrine system, and the often-quoted truism that it takes seven years to replace all the cells of the body[65].

Apart from physical health, we see the Rule of Seven at work in the development of the individual. Every seven years puts us in a new cycle of growth. The years one to seven are marked by infancy and then rudimentary learning. The next seven years are the true childhood years, ending with adolescence and the beginning of the physical maturing process. At the end of the next seven-year cycle, the individual has achieved adulthood. Young adulthood is experienced for the next seven years, and it is in the fourth cycle—from the age of twenty-eight to thirty-five—that we typically become the essence of who we will be for the rest of our lives. Some call this the "construction" phase, where people acquire possessions and property, typically establishing a home and family. This is further developed in

---

[65] This controversial "law" has been refuted and supposedly disproved, however more recent experiments have affirmed that most, if not all, the cells of the body are replaced in a period of as little as five years, but not longer than seven years, depending on genetically inherited metabolic characteristics. So this particular "Rule of Seven" is essentially valid even if not always literally and precisely true.

the next seven years, which end at age 42 and from there we pass into the next cycle, usually referred to as "middle age". This is when reassessment usually takes place, preparing the individual for starting a new cycle of sevens as the fiftieth year approaches.

As you can see, there are distinct characteristics of each seven-year period in the average person's life, even though there is no actual delineation of the periods. We go through life growing and changing gradually, and the periods are seamless. It is only when one stops to examine a life in total that certain patterns appear.

Rudolph Steiner, the father of Anthroposophical medicine, also invoked the Rule of Seven and said that seven-year cycles are an important aspect of not only physical health but mental development and the social sciences as well.

Most have heard of the *Sirocco*, a wind in the northern Mediterranean that blows in from the Sahara desert that is associated with negative changes in personality and behavior in people. In fact, the justice system is known to be lenient in sentencing people who commit crimes during this period because of the uncharacteristic changes in their personalities. Switzerland has a similar warm, dry air current traditionally called "the Evil Wind". The *Foehn* is observed to always coincide with a sharp uptick in violent crime.

Since oxygen can hold positive and negative charges, medical climatologists have studied the effects of negative and positive ionization and have found that changes in human behavior can correlate with subtle changes in the air. The Nobel Prize-winning Swedish scientist Svante Arrhenius (originator of the "greenhouse effect" theory) proved that ion conductivity in the atmosphere coincided with a dramatic increase in crime, and that some of these changes occur predictably every 27.5 days. The half day notwithstanding, this is roughly a pattern of 7 x 4.

Haven't you noticed that at some point your hair began to behave differently? If you asked your barber or hairdresser why, you were probably told (as I was) that the hair patterns change every seven years.

Most animals have a lifespan of seven times the period of maturity. For example, a dog matures within two years, and lives (depending on the breed) twelve to fourteen years. For that reason, many naturopathic writers (including Uncle Earl) have speculated that the natural life span of a human being should be 140 years, if following Nature's laws of health. It's a nice theory, but *not one* of even the most impeccable figures in natural medicine has ever lasted so long[66].

All this is being mentioned not to insist that everything follows an immutable law of sevens; there are certainly plenty of natural cycles that do not follow multiples of that number. *But the distinct differences in the development periods of both the personality and the human body are replicated in the development of illness:* There are infancy, childhood, middle age, and old age periods of chronic diseases, so to speak. It is our intent to point out that therapeutic measures must be adapted to the period of the illness, in the same way that communication with a seven year old must of necessity be different from that of a fourteen year old. The measures that would be effective in the early stages of an illness are not indicated when it is advanced, and vice-versa.

To return to Lindlahr's Rule of Seven, elucidated by the author's uncle: It is typical to see patients who have commenced treatment (whether it is by oral medicines or physical therapies, detoxification or diet) experience *either improvement or worsening in seven days.* The worsening of symptoms (the classic "aggravation", "healing crisis", or "re-tracing", depending on your vocabulary), if it occurs, is generally followed by improvement, which then continues over a period of time. At seven weeks, the patient very

---

[66] Including Uncle Earl, who only made it to 98,(although it took a head injury to do it).

predictably has a relapse. If treatment is accurate for the stage of healing that the patient is now in, improvement will again occur and if the problem seems mostly resolved, you can plan on seeing the patient again at about the seven month mark, when he will claim, "It's starting to come back." Or it may be a "new" problem that brings him in, but if it is occurring at the seventh month, it is likely that it is not really a "new" problem at all, but one that was deeper and hidden before. The clearing of the original complaints allowed the older and deeper problem to emerge, which was asymptomatic before.

I have seen this scenario played out countless times in forty three years of practice. It is relevant, not because it is a part of traditional naturopathic teachings, but because it is a repeatedly observable phenomenon. On those occasions when the Rule of Seven is taken into consideration, the treatment plan typically bears good fruit. The results are invariably disappointing, however, when I have been (1) pressed for time and simply repeated the same treatment or prescription at a different stage of healing, or (2) administered a particular treatment at the insistence of the patient, rather than a more accurate one, or (3) treated out of the proper sequence, or (4) over-treated in an attempt to better insure good results. The correct counterparts to these shortcomings will become more clearly explained in the last section of this book.

It is our intent to point out that therapeutic measures must be adapted to the period of the illness, in the same way that communication with a seven year old must of necessity be different from that of a fourteen year old.

Bowen Therapy, as referred to previously, creates therapeutic changes that develop over seven days' time. Those receiving Bowen treatment are advised to not have any therapy (including further Bowen treatment) during that seven-day period, as it tends to interfere with the full development of the therapeutic results of the previous Bowen session.

Before my naturopathic training, and before my training in Oriental medicine, I was a shiatsu therapist. My Japanese shiatsu teacher taught me to press the points for seven seconds. No explanation was ever given for this, aside from a vague statement that it took that length of time for the point to "become active". "Count to ten," he said, "For most people counting that will be seven seconds." So I mentally counted to ten many thousands of times as I applied acupressure, until the duration of time was instinctive and did not require counting.

The admonition "Count to ten" was remembered, but only now do I recall that the points were actually stimulated for *seven* seconds.

During my study of classical acupuncture, I learned that the legendary Hua Tuo applied moxibustion to points in *seven* increments, allowing that number of moxa cones to burn on a point.

Later, during studies in German electro-acupuncture, we learned that many exciting discoveries were being made in Europe that further developed the therapies from the Far East. In particular, German scientists researching acupuncture discovered that within the traditionally-held time parameters for the circulation of bioelectrical energy in the human body, there existed smaller cycles within the same time periods. By monitoring these minute changes in amplitude and polarity of electricity in the human body, it was found that changes occurred in rhythmic cycles of just over seven minutes. They termed this period a "*khroe*". The effects of electro-acupuncture could be more predictable by timing the stimulation to match with the appropriate phase of electrical activity.

In the 1920s, a man named Harvey Spencer Lewis wrote a book called *Self Mastery and Fate with the Cycles of Life.* Lewis was a resoundingly successful businessman who used a system on which to base business decisions and activities. Railroad magnate Arthur Stilwell said of Lewis: "H. Spencer

Lewis has been the real 'silent partner' and secret adviser in more big business propositions in America than any other living man." Lewis wrote the book detailing his system after retiring from business life. The system, as the reader probably suspects, is based on cycles of seven.

In his book, Lewis describes the changes in the developing individual and the characteristics of each phase of seven years, as has been mentioned here. He then divides the calendar year into seven periods of fifty-two days each. In calculating the periods from the birth date, he finds that natural cycles exist that make certain actions more auspicious in one than another. Additionally, when a business is viewed in the same way, the different periods in the course of a year present very definitive aspects. In one period, advertising is most effective. In a different period, it will not be. In certain of the periods, expansion is advised; in another, it is not. Lewis maintains that there are advantageous times for securing loans, renewing contracts, etc.—based on there being seven distinct periods in a year. Each day, also, can be divided into seven periods, each of which has beneficial and negative aspects. Timing one's actions to the proper time period, according to Lewis, leads to success in one's undertakings. However cosmically significant you may think this is or is not, remember that Lewis made millions for himself and others using his system.

You will recall that the mortality doubling time, an age-related milestone that doubles the likelihood of one's dying, increases every seven to eight years.

At this point the reader may think the author is dizzily seeing sevens everywhere he looks, but explain this: In conventional medical thinking, an acute condition is considered to become chronic when it lasts for more than six months. Why does an illness become chronic from the **seventh month** onward?[67]

[67] Although when I was in school we were taught that a condition becomes subacute at 3 months and chronic at 6, it is now the convention in mainstream medicine to call something "chronic" at 3 months' duration.

A clinician of any type will recognize that cycles of acute illness are different from chronic illness, and will require different treatment. We can visualize acute illness as having a "short wave length", in electronic terms. Fluctuations in symptoms, fever, discharge, etc., will occur often, as expressed in the illustration. One does not need to point out that **the typical acute illness lasts an average of seven days** (unless treated inappropriately, in which case it lingers or changes its symptoms). If untreated, it usually lasts a week, which the reader has undoubtedly observed.

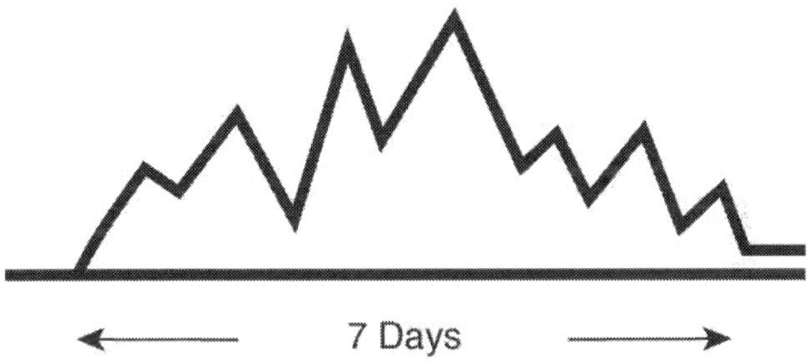

In terms of medicine, dosing in such a case needs to be aggressive; the medicine needs to be repeated more often than if the illness is subacute or chronic, because the virulence of the illness often demands it.

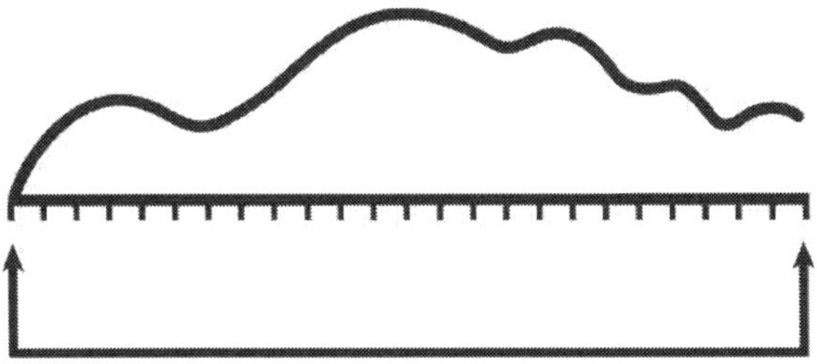

ACUTE: 24 hour period with symptoms varying in intensity

Medicine taken frequently…

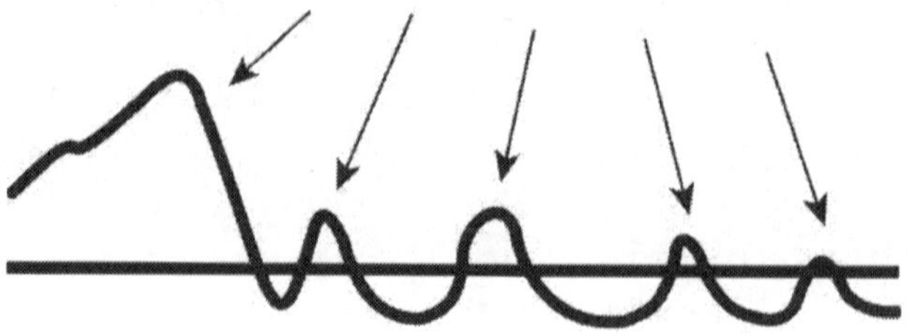

… repeatedly pushes illness down

As we can see from the illustration, applying medicine or treatment just as the symptoms begin to rise again acts to prevent the process from returning to its peak, and can result in a slower and weaker impulse to relapse. Intervention may need to be hourly in the beginning, then less often as the disease process becomes less aggressive.

Chronic illnesses, on the other hand, can be seen to be a "long wave", and will tend to have exacerbations or remissions at greater intervals. These very often occur at the seventh month.

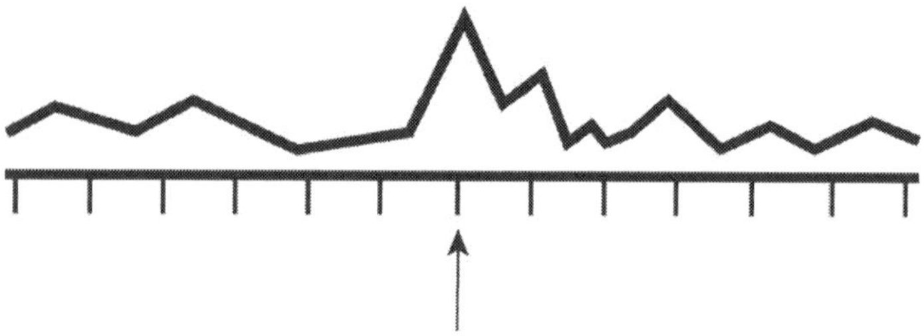

Flare-up at 7th month

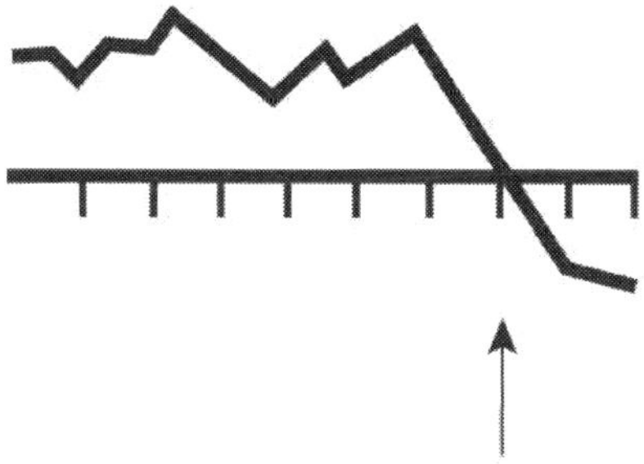

Remission at 7th month

In such a case, periodic doses of medicine are preferred. If timed appropriately, a healing response can be activated at the point when the body is most susceptible to the imprint of new information. If treatment or medication is followed unchangingly throughout the natural cycles, however, it overrides the inclination on the part of the body to correct the problem, and this approach is the "suppressive treatment" that is warned against in natural medicine.

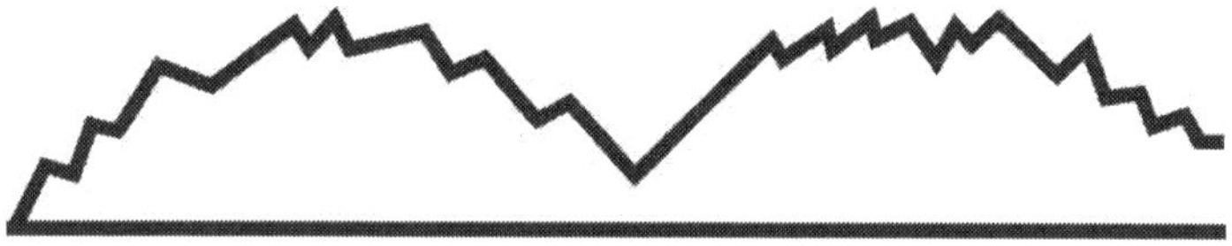

CHRONIC: 7 weeks of building, then receding, symptoms. Cycle begins again after seven weeks.

Patterns in diet and allergy follow the same laws: Desensitizing someone to a food trigger usually requires abstinence from the offending food for 6 weeks, re-introducing it into the diet at the 7th week and allowing days to pass before eating it again. **Week 7 is the critical point for re-introduction, just as resting periods between the stimulations are essential** (like those used in Bowen Therapy).

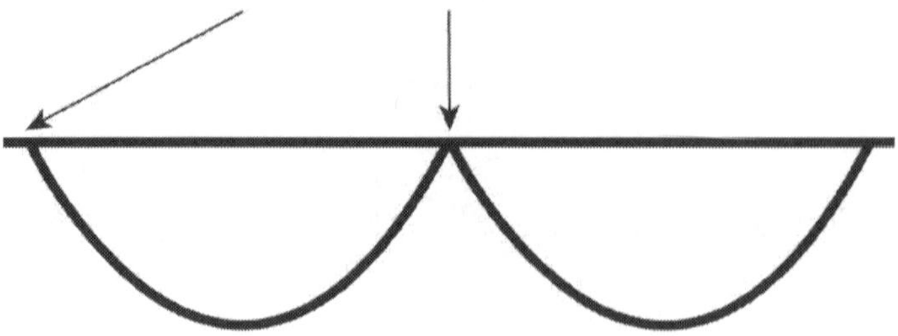

TREATMENT CAUSES OPPOSITE WAVE:
Condition begins to recur at the 7th week; re-treating causes it to recede again.

Unconscious use of the Rule of Seven and Bowen-discovered principles are common in medicine. The author has made no new discovery here. The Septimal Law is simply his rendering of a widely-observed natural rhythm that can enhance the reader's efforts if care is taken to scrutinize, and carefully apply treatment at the most advantageous time.

ACUTE ILLNESS

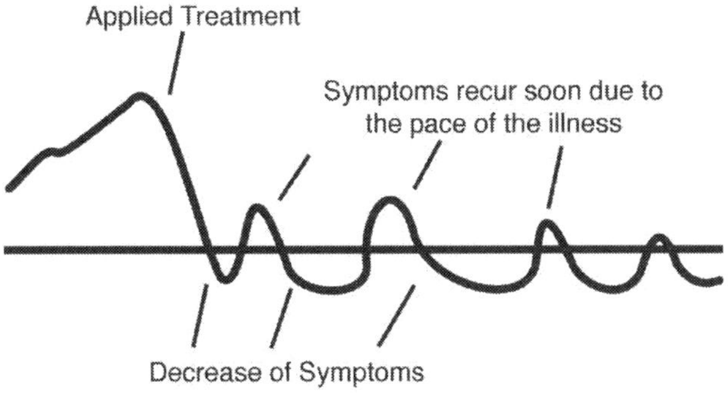

Acute illnesses require a more aggressive approach, and a more frequent repetition of oral medicine or hands-on therapy, as the case may be. Since the symptoms undulate at a rapid rate (i.e., every few hours rather than days), treatment must match the pace of the illness, decreasing when the body requires less aid.

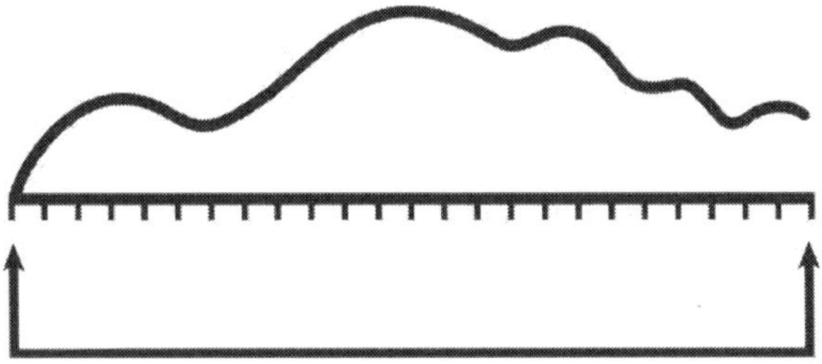

ACUTE: 24 hour period with symptoms varying in intensity

CHRONIC ILLNESS

In a chronic illness, symptoms are slower to develop, fluctuate less often, and require periodic (rather than continuous and aggressive) treatment in order to effectively change the pattern of behavior on the part of the body (or mind). Within a few repetitions of the therapy, remission will be observed to last longer and longer periods of time—unless interfered with by too frequent or ill-timed sessions or dosing.

CHRONIC ILLNESS

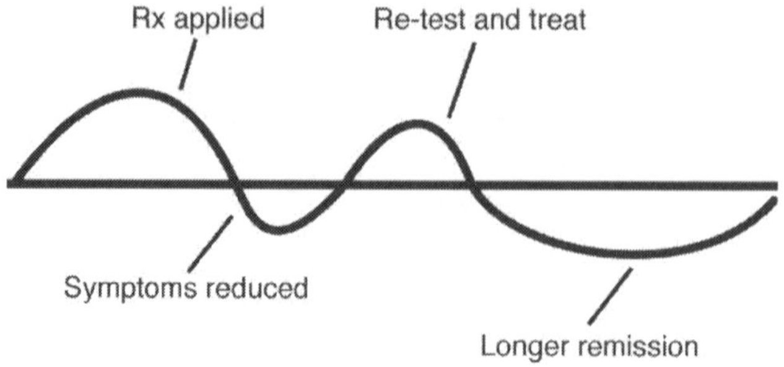

It should occur to the reader that the emphasis on acute care and symptomatic treatment is the reason conventional allopathic medicine has the stronger reputation compared to gentler methods typically grouped under the diplomatic heading of “wellness”. As stated here, acute illnesses require a more aggressive approach—and allopathic therapeutics are more easily applied in a peremptory manner. Simply being able to apply remedies intravenously, and thereby obviating the need to wait for the body to absorb and process a reaction, gives mainstream medicine a great advantage in controlling emergent conditions.[68]

Allopathic medicine’s track record on chronic diseases, however, is not as impressive. This is the reason so many people turn to “alternative” methods to resolve their longstanding problems. Illnesses that developed over time and have been present for a time respond best to therapies that, like the problems themselves, take time. Thus, you see practitioners of all stripes slowly and gently improving their patients’ health with non-mainstream methods.

---

[68] Even so, once I recognized the principles in Uni-Syn, I was better able to apply the various naturopathic, homeopathic, botanical, acupuncture, and manual therapies I already used, with the result that I am much more effective in treating acute illness than I had been in the past, even using the same treatments.

The Septimal Law in Applying the Principle of Periodicity

Acupuncture treatment for chronic conditions is typically done daily in the Far East; however, in the West treatments are more often applied weekly. A seven-day cycle has been adopted due to economic and cultural differences, but it is the author's suspicion that unconscious use of the Rule of Seven may be something that has been instinctively worked out in order to boost effectiveness. Of course, it also may be because acupuncturists are mostly treating chronic conditions.

If one examines a seven-day interval of treatment superimposed against the natural cycling of the patient's symptoms, it becomes more clear:

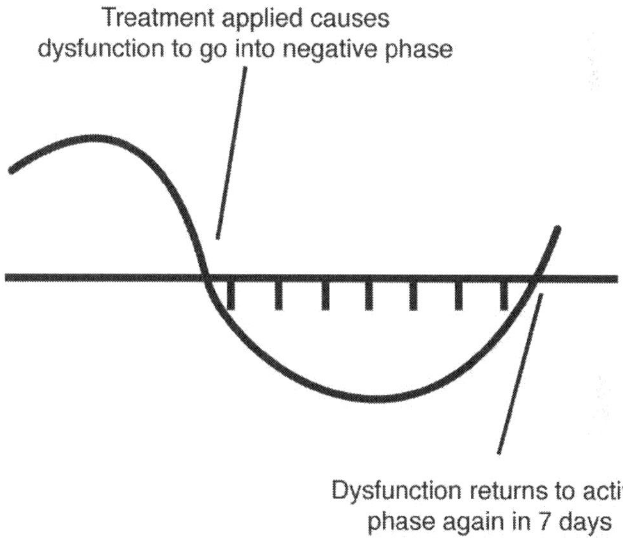

This applies to subacute conditions, and the beginning of treatment for chronic cases. It does not apply to acute conditions, of course, for obvious reasons. But a not-so-obvious reason is that acute conditions are better served with a seven-hour interval or a three-and-a-half hour interval. A treatment applied at the seven-hour mark will surprisingly manage symptoms quite well (although this is not possible to achieve in the clinic; home procedures are applied). Symptoms of greater intensity will be managed by therapy every 3½ hours (half of seven). It may be that the pharmaceuticals that are often dosed every four hours are using this principle inadvertently. The author has heard many stories from patients who have said "I could tell when it was time to take the medicine again!" The fact that the drug "wore off" before the four hours was up suggests that something closer to a 3½ hour cycle was involved. Medicine dosed every eight hours usually finds the patient feeling not so well in the last hour before taking the medicine again—the victim of a seven-hour cycle passing into the active phase again.

Now consider the patient with a chronic condition, treated effectively with some therapy such as acupuncture, Chiropractic, Bowen Therapy, etc. Visualize the diminishing amplitude of the patient's symptoms as he or she undergoes a weekly treatment regimen:

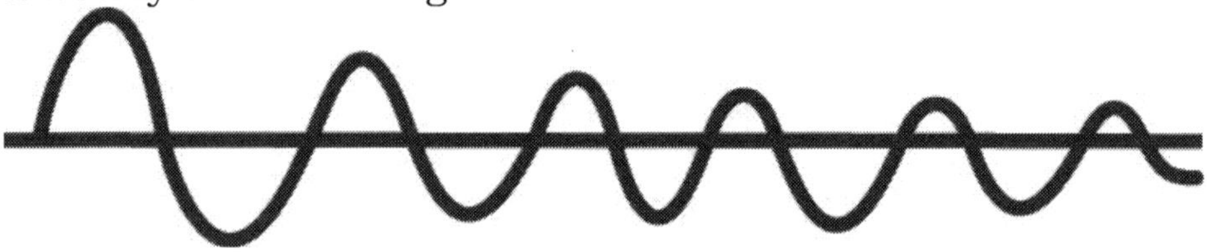

As the patient's body cycles through, the treatment is applied each time the cycle causes the symptoms to try to rebound (usually at the seventh day). Gradually, the process becomes weakened and the amplitude of the illness diminishes as it passes through successive rounds of weekly therapy.

It should be noted that Bowen Therapy insists on weekly sessions with *no* intercurrent therapy or stimulation, as it is felt that any additional stimulation while the body is producing the seven-day response to the treatment will be counter-productive. It appears that Bowen Therapy is clearly taking advantage of the Septimal Law.

Duration of Therapy Session

As for the individual treatment sessions themselves, it is established in most physical therapies that a twenty-minute application is the most effective. Exercise physiologists insist on maintaining target heart rate range for a period of twenty minutes for an effective session. Whether it is rehabilitation or physical therapy, electrical stimulation, hydrotherapy, infrared, diathermy, or other modalities, peak effectiveness in twenty minutes has been observed. Even in acupuncture, the twenty-minute mark has been shown to deliver the maximum response, as noted by celebrated experts such as acupuncturist Dr. Giovanni Maciocia.

Since any practitioner can tell you that one seldom returns to the patient in order to discontinue the therapy exactly as the twenty-minute timer goes off, it is likely that a good part of the time, patients are actually receiving 21-minute treatments, or at least close to it. *What if the optimal period of stimulation (or exercise, etc.) was 21 minutes?* Let us examine the periodicity of that time spent under treatment.

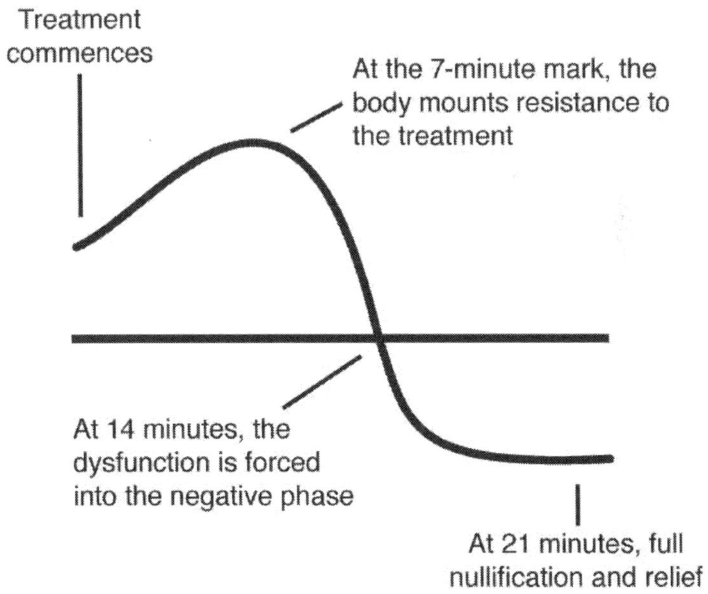

In applying oral medicines, it has long been the author's method when treating chronic conditions to dose for three weeks at a time, followed by one week's rest, before returning for follow-up consultation at the fourth week. With a chronic illness, there will typically be cyclical changes at seven-day intervals; we simply work with the cycles.

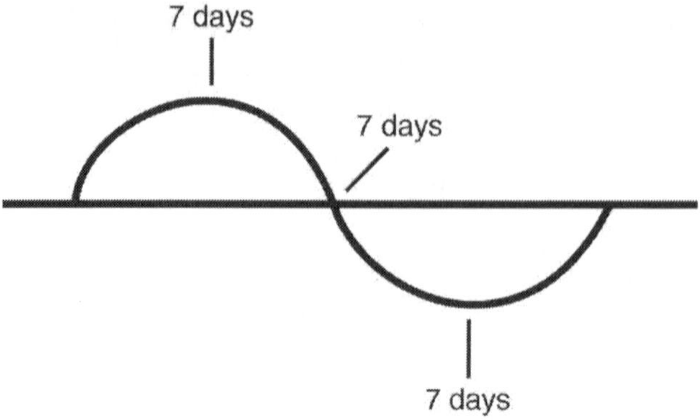

A 21-day cycle of therapy, putting the illness in a different phase at 21 days.

At the follow-up consultation at the four-week mark, it will usually be obvious if the prescription needs to be repeated or changed, or if (more often than not) no action is needed at all. The 21-day course of medicine, if it has produced some momentum in healing, will be continuing to act and the patient will still be improved. If, however, the patient was better while taking the agent but began to relapse in the last few days after discontinuing, then the practitioner knows that a higher potency, or a longer course of the same potency, is needed.

It may have occurred to the reader that the period of isolation for those exposed to virulent contagious diseases (e.g., Ebola virus) is 21 days. Public health authorities consider the three-week period as ideal for observation as to whether a person has been infected or are contagious themselves. This makes sense in light of what we know about the Septimal Law and the Polarity principle, for three weeks allows the disease process time to go from visibility to dormancy and back again (or positive up phase to positive down phase to negative phase).

Since most practitioners of the types referred to in this book routinely treat musculoskeletal conditions, a final example of this aspect of periodicity will be given.

Most authoritative sources in orthopedic medicine advise rest for the treatment of tendonitis and synovitis, *for a period of three weeks* (21 days, 3 x 7). This allows the tendon to heal, the synovial membranes to stop the inflammatory cycle, and the condition to resolve. The Septimal Law is once again unknowingly invoked.

This is mentioned to illustrate that it is not only the invisible workings of the acupuncture meridians, or the "innate intelligence" of the body from the chiropractic viewpoint, the "vis" of naturopathic philosophy, or the "vital force" of the homeopathic framework that are affected by these cycles. Gross pathologies, objective tissue changes—*conventionally defined diseases*—are subject to these laws.

> "The lunar month has such special power over our bodies that not only births, but diseases, death or recovery have a kind of dependence on such revolution."
>
> —-Hippocrates

15

THE LAWS OF MINIMIZATION

Less is more.

(Buddhist maxim)

In addition to the "Three Ps", there are two other important principles that govern effective therapy, Minimization and Detachment, covered in this and the following chapters.

The first principle to complement the preceding three laws is expressed best in the ancient Buddhist admonition: "Less is more".

Hua Tuo, the venerable master acupuncturist whose discoveries were mentioned with regard to the vertebral points, also contributed to the understanding of "less is more".

When Hua Tuo performed acupuncture, it was in only one or two places. As he inserted the needle, he would instruct the patient to tell him when he felt a sensation at a distant area, saying that he was going to mentally direct the energy there. When the patient told him that the sensation reached the target area, Hua Tuo would withdraw the needle. He reputedly had great success with this method.[69]

As mentioned earlier: If Hua Tuo employed moxibustion, he would only burn the moxa in one or two places and in each

[69] DeWoskin, Kenneth J., *Doctors, Diviners and Magicians of Ancient China: Biographies of Fang-Shih.* 1983 Columbia University Press.

location he reportedly burned seven cones of moxa. Thus, the point would be stimulated specifically seven times, whereas usually the number of stimulations was based on whether the point was being tonified or sedated.

So once again we have the Septimal Law or "Rule of Seven" being invoked, as well as the minimalist approach to provocation.

Prof. G. Kellner of the University of Vienna, whose research into acupuncture in the 1960s is legendary, found that even small punctures would affect the body neurologically for at least five days.

The "minimum dose" in Homeopathy is one obvious example of minimalist methodology. Another is the "drop dose" prescribing of the Eclectic physicians (a quantity of a fluid extract stirred into a glass of water and teaspoon doses of the mixture taken).

A more modern treatment method, Low Level Laser Therapy, has been researched to reveal very critical dosage schedules. Laser strength of 8 to 16 joules/cm_2 is effective for pain reduction, but a lower concentration at 0.5 to 5 joules/cm_2 will initiate tissue repair. Once again, while moderate doses inhibit (as per the Arndt-Schultz Law), small doses are needed to actually promote healing, as opposed to clearing pathological processes.

Thyroid hormones, present in the blood in a minimal concentration of only one fifty-millionth, control your metabolism. Less is more.

How many parts per million does the concentration of pollen in the air have to be in order to provoke an allergic reaction?

Interestingly, hypnotized subjects told that they have an allergy to corn, then given it to eat, have manifested the same IgE antibody formations and exhibited the same allergic symptoms as those truly allergic to corn. The allergic reaction is not "imaginary", but the mechanism is as immaterial or minimal as anything could be. In other words, even *infinitely* less is more.

Minimalist Massage

A study was conducted at Cedars-Sinai Medical Center in Los Angeles investigating the biochemical effects of massage. The project was sponsored by the National Center for Complementary and Alternative Medicine (a division of the National Institutes of Health). Researchers took 53 healthy adults and randomly assigned 29 of them to a 45-minute session of deep-tissue Swedish massage and the other 24 to a session of light massage.

Subjects were fitted with intravenous catheters so that blood samples could be taken immediately before the massage and at various times up to an hour after.

The volunteers who received Swedish massage experienced significant decreases in levels of the "stress hormone" cortisol in both blood and saliva samplings. Also levels of amino acid l-arginine and vasopressin (a hormone that can lead to increases in cortisol) were reduced. As in other studies of massage benefits, the subjects had increases in their lymphocyte count, showing positive immune system effects.

Subjects who had the light massage evidenced greater increases in oxytocin, a hormone associated with contentment, than the Swedish massage group, and a larger release of cortisol than the deep massage group.

The extended deep massage can be said to have created a sedation effect; one in which the biochemical components that create increased organic and neuromotor activity are reduced. Or, in the traditional language of acupuncture, an excess has been dispersed.

The light massage can be said to have created a tonifying effect, where the elements needed for increased activity are stimulated. An increased release of cortisol powers the body to new heights of activity. Interestingly, the release of oxytocin seems to counterbalance the stress-inducing effects of the cortisol release.

It goes without saying that light massage is performed with less effort expended on the part of the therapist.

Original (minimalist) Principles of Osteopathy

In Dr. Still's original conception, the body was seen to be a complete unit in which no individual part works in isolation. It is a self-regulating organism that has (in today's parlance) a "default programming" of healing, whenever dysfunction occurs. In order for this to be achieved, Still taught that there must be integrity of the nervous system and the vascular system. Correcting the "lesions" that impinge on these systems, as we learned in Chapter Two, became the goal of the osteopathic manipulation.

So far, this establishes the rationale for just about every system that considers itself "holistic". But a key principle of early Osteopathy is the concept of the "primary lesion"—the loss of mobility and function that the other dysfunctions in the patient stem from. The traditional osteopath learned to find the most critical location(s)[70] to apply treatment in the same way that a bowler tries to hit the pin that will knock down all the others.

The principle of "less is more" was certainly a part of original Osteopathy.

[70] The chiropractor refers to these as "majors".

There is also a famous quote by B.J. Palmer, the major developer of the Chiropractic profession, that echoes this concept. I am told that this aphorism hung on the wall of Palmer College of Chiropractic in Davenport, Iowa:

> The fundamental of this clinic is to see ***how little*** we can do, at ***how few places***, ***how rarely***, and ***how quickly*** it can be done, to accomplish the ***greatest change*** in the ***shortest space of time***, at the ***least*** cost to the case, and to know ***what*** to do and ***why*** we do it, ***before*** doing it.
>
> —B.J. Palmer

If this is not the wisest advice for *any* type of health care practitioner, I don't know what would be. It certainly gives us more specific guidance than the Hippocratic dictum *Primum non nocere* ("First, do no harm").

Exercise and Minimization

I was trying to build my physique with free weights as a teenager in the 1960s, and was having mixed success when I stumbled upon a bodybuilding "gadget". It consisted of a metal plate with a hasp in the middle. Through the hasp ran a rope, connected on the other end to a handlebar. There was a series of exercises to be done by standing on the plate, gripping the handlebar, and pulling against the rope in various positions and angles. This device, referred to as a "minute-a-day gym", did in fact require only a minute to perform all the exercises, because—amazingly—they required only two seconds of effort each.

The secret was isometric contraction, and the literature that came with the device referenced studies done at Max Planck Institute in Germany and George Williams College in the

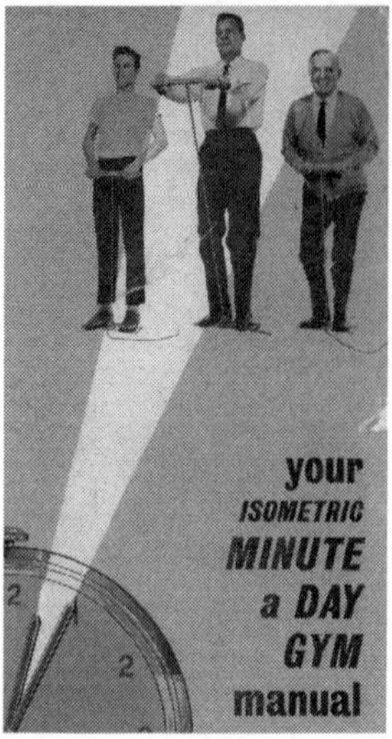

U.S.A. showing that muscles that had maximum stimulation (as in straining at the maximum of effort) were unresponsive to any further stimulation that day. This too-good-to-be-true revelation certainly proved valid in my case, because I experienced great advances in my muscular development; far more from the "one minute" I spent with this device daily than with the dozens of repetitions I had formerly been doing with weights[71].

Exercise and fitness theory has been dominated since the 1970s by the *aerobic* model. This means medium-intensity, high-volume exercise, in the form of running, treadmill, rowing machines, and lots of non-stop calisthenics. Exercise is done for an extended period of time, but only at a moderate intensity.

The opposite of this is a high-intensity, low-volume workout, where you would use almost all your strength or speed, but for only a short period of time, followed by rest or low activity. This is called *interval* training, and this model is now being endorsed for athletic competition for its ability to enhance sports performance. **Such is an example of how Minimization is possible because of Periodicity.**

A study comparing the two models revealed that interval training improved athletic performance and cardiac function far beyond continuous aerobic exercise[72]. Non-stop aerobic activity, the classic "cardiopulmonary exercise", was not only ineffective in enhancing sports performance, but showed itself to be much less effective in improving cardiac function.

---

[71] The reader should now realize that the typical weight lifting practice of doing 10-12 repetitions in three "sets" interspersed with rest periods invokes the Law of Periodicity. Doing thirty straight repetitions does not produce the same result.

[72] Meyer, et al., *Interval Vs. Continuous Exercise Training After Coronary Bypass Surgery: A Comparison of Training-Induced Acute Reactions With Respect to the Effectiveness of the Exercise Methods*, Clin Cardiol, Dec. 1990.

The study was done, by the way, with patients who had already had coronary bypass surgery.

Another study using peak oxygen volume monitoring also found that interval training was superior to non-stop exercise.[73] Yet another study used comprehensive measuring of blood volume, oxygen volume, and the heart's ventricular strength, and showed that brief, high-intensity training is 2½ times as effective in improving cardiovascular function as non-stop medium-level exercise[74].

There was another published study that showed that endurance training actually made the heart *weaker!* [75] But the "gold standard" for exercise in many people's minds continues to be endurance training, like running, treadmill, etc. Physicians warn patients, particularly heart patients, about high-intensity exercise and steer them toward aerobics.

And most recently, a 25-year study was concluded by researchers at Kaiser Permanente that showed that those who exercised far beyond the national guidelines of 150 minutes exercise weekly were 86% more likely to develop coronary artery calcifications by middle age[76].

I've gone on about this more than I intended, but I think it is an important point that **science says strength training makes the heart stronger, and "cardio" training weakens it.**[77] The exercise methods most often touted as "scientific"

---

[73] Rugnmo, et al., *High Intensity Aerobic Interval Exercise Is Superior To Moderate Intensity Exercise For Increasing Aerobic Capacity In Patients With Coronary Artery Disease,* Eur J Cardiovasc Prev Rehabil, June 2004.

[74] Warburton, et al., *Blood Volume Expansion And Cardio Respiratory Function: Effects Of Training Modality*, Med Sci Sports Exerc. June 2004.

[75] Delagardelle, et al., *Strength/Endurance Training Vs. Endurance Training In Congestive Heart Failure,* Med Sci Sports Exerc. Dec. 2002.

[76] DOI: http://dx.doi.org/10.1016/j.mayocp.2017.07.016

[77] More information on this topic is covered in another book, *The Negri Manual of Natural Medicine.*

are therefore actually not very scientific, and not greatly achieving what the people performing them desired in the first place. But with a high-intensity, short duration exercise, less is spent and more is achieved. Read that: "Less is more".

This is why the drills seen in Asian martial arts traditionally last only a minute or so. The *kata* of karate, stick fighting, fencing, etc., are brief, dynamic exercises. The various forms of yoga also hold their postures for only brief periods, moving on to different positions in a minute or two. The effort is not maintained all that long. And remember that these activities were set down centuries before anyone ever did a study of "interval training".

The action that appears to be the purpose of the activity—lifting weights, holding a yoga pose, stimulating an acupuncture point, taking a medicine, manipulating a joint, etc.—is nothing without its invisible counterbalancing-and-developing rest period.

Even the long-followed dictum of performing multiple sets of an exercise in weight lifting has been shown by research to be unnecessary, and was published by the Journal of Exercise Physiology[78]. Multiple sets do not contribute substantially to muscular development as was previously thought. But it should be pointed out that they do contribute substantially to the time and effort expended in gaining the benefits of exercise. Minimization as a principle, while easily tested, is contrary to long-held dogma and is not likely to result in a revision of methods that have shaped our expectations for generations. But it is nevertheless true.

[78] http://ssudl.solent.ac.uk/2274

Bone Density: Provocation, Polarity, Periodicity ...and Minimization

A study[79] at the University of Bristol in England tested young women who repeatedly jumped off and back onto a box 15 inches high. They hopped ten times, *pausing 30 seconds between hops*, twice daily. They showed significant gains in hip bone density after four months. Another group that hopped twenty times instead of ten showed even greater gains. The rest times between jumps, it seems, is necessary (which we understand by now, by a study of the Law of Periodicity). The shock generated by the impact with the ground provided the provocation, the ions being displaced in the bone (piezoelectric effect) provided the polarity, the rest time provided the periodicity. Altogether, it represents a minimization of effort for a good return. Improved bone density for ten hops? A good return on investment in anyone's book.

Weight Loss Through Minimization

General fitness is not the only category where this surprising fact has relevance. It is just as applicable to weight loss. The September 2013 issue of the *American Journal of Health Promotion* reports on a study done at the University of Utah. They found that brief sessions of intense exercise created as much, if not more, weight loss than moderate-level, sustained activity of ten minutes or more. It was noted that adding just one minute of vigorous activity to a typical subject's day caused a half-pound difference in weight compared to a control group.

The "one minute a day", which seemed like an adman's lie when it described my exercise device, now shows measurable weight loss.

---

[79] Hardcastle, SA, Gregson, CL, Rittweger, J, Crabtree, N, Ward, K & Tobias, JH 2014, *Jump power and force have distinct associations with cortical bone parameters: Findings from a population enriched by individuals with high bone mass.* Journal of Clinical Endocrinology and Metabolism, vol 99., pp. 266-275

Steady, unchanging aerobic exercise works initially to help one lose weight, but then the body adapts and starts to conserve energy; fat burning declines. In other words, the effects of the activity within the body *begin to change polarity.* This is the reason for including this information here.

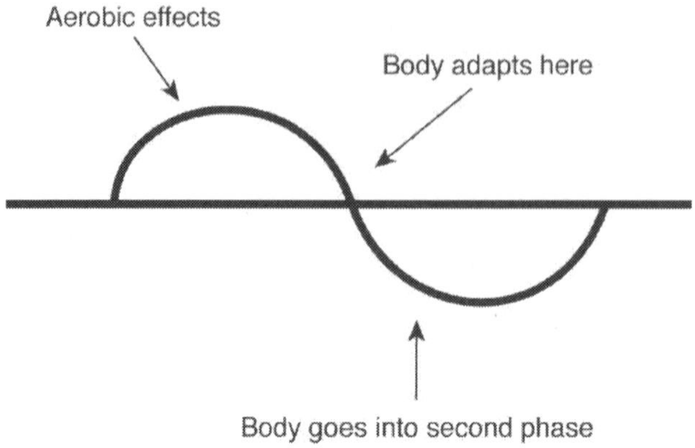

Raising the metabolic rate and increasing fat burning is really achieved by varying the exercise: a fast pace for a few minutes, then increasing resistance by moving uphill, etc., then going slower downhill, then integrating weight lifting, etc. This is defined as "interval training", referred to earlier. This will give residual fat-burning potential for hours after the activity. Why?

It can be seen that all of this is nothing more than another illustration of the Polarity Principle. Reducing the intensity of the exercise, or changing its focus, before the body can adapt and produce a Phase Two response (which creates the opposite effects), one can maintain only the action desired. This can be illustrated in this way:

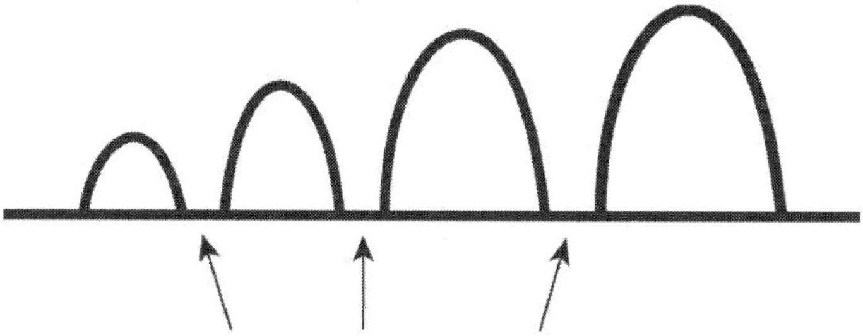

Intervals with changing activity leads to increasing gains before 2nd phase can occur

Why is this not more widely recognized?[80]

Now, all these years after using my little mail order muscle-building tool, I have more insight into the nature of this mysterious principle that created its effects, but also more insight into the complex social and commercial reasons that we are often not aware of such facts.

Should we be surprised that so many discoveries and good ideas are buried? What happens to all the complex (and expensive) exercise machines, all the free weights, all the gymnasiums and health centers with trainers if a little handlebar/rope/foot plate gizmo was in every home? Of course, that simple device cannot produce all the effects that can be had from a variety of exercise equipment, but it could replace many of them.

Therc are tremendous commercial pressures to maintain the status quo—in every field—even to the extent that methods that do not produce the best results are mainstream while the best methods are obscure (or even discredited). Readers with an insight into medical politics know this well. Those methods that are most effective are the most ruthlessly suppressed. Non-drug therapies that threaten

[80] In medicine, when public pressure demands a stand on a method that is unpopular with the orthodox medical community, studies are done that "prove" that the method is ineffective. The widely-circulated articles mocking homeopathic medicine are good examples, or the "study" that Vitamin E can be harmful. The de-bunking studies are always more publicized than the quality trials that show that the method actually works.

pharmaceutical industry profits have historically been attacked.

The simple, sad fact is this: The methods that become mainstream are those that produce *some* improvement, but not cure. This insures long-term treatment. Moreover, they must produce—and here is the insidious part—*side effects.* There must be a downside to the therapy or activity that causes another problem, for which another therapy or medicine is needed.

In the pharmaceutical industry, a drug in development that shows little to no toxicity will be discarded (or as an industry insider once told me, "It goes in File 13").[81]

Making all this possible is one of the simplest tasks of applied psychology. What reasonable physician is going to believe that something that grows in her backyard can rival a potent drug manufactured by an FDA-approved laboratory? What athlete who has spent countless hours doing countless repetitions with free weights and cam-driven exercise machines is going to believe that his muscular development could have been gained from a minute's effort?

Isometric exercise is not the only kind of exercise we need, of course. But the story of my little device illustrates the startling results that can sometimes be gained from a minimum of effort and time, and that is what Uni-Syn represents in the world of therapy.

Now that we have examined why the principle of minimum stimulation is important, it is also important (to me) to point out that, in all honesty, I have violated this rule many times. In fact, most of us have; when we are doubtful about how complete a patient's relief is going to be at the end of the treatment, we add a bit extra as insurance. If we really like the patient, we add a bit extra. If we are afraid of losing the

---

[81] So it is with many fields, and explains the absence of the 100-mile-per-gallon carburetor, the free wireless electric power of Nikola Tesla, and numerous other inventions that would have made life better at the expense of big business.

patient due to slow progress, we add. And if we allow the patient to bully us into treating everything under the sun in one session, we do likewise. It is nearly always a mistake. Even the Collins General Naturopathic Tonic Technique, which I have delivered many times and love doing, is too much treatment for the average case—and it only takes five minutes to perform. But it can be overkill.

Why? Let me ask you this: What if eight people surrounded you and all talked to you at the same time? How would your brain handle it? Would you process what each one was saying? How much would you take away from the conversation? And what would your level of stress be? Personally, I would short circuit.

The brain of the patient must register clearly the stimulation that you are creating with your treatment. Chiropractic research has shown that if only one or two spinal segments are adjusted, the patient responds well because there is no confusion in the nervous system. The neurological change is made, and the patient regains balance.

What happens if we manipulate eight segments in the spine, or needle twenty acupuncture points, or massage every reflex point? The body would be confused. This is why less is more.

Another aspect of this, by the way, is financial. A patient whose response to treatment is muddled will drift away from your practice. A patient who is seen for a short time and given a to-the-point treatment that seems decisive will respond better—and they will refer others. Most people will get somewhat better, regardless of the treatment. But the patient who is impressed with you will refer. Food for thought.

16

THE LAWS OF DETACHMENT

The final invisible but necessary element in effective healing is the practice of Detachment. Now we are in the realm of immeasurable forces that nonetheless have a profound impact on the quality of any therapy administered to a patient.

We are not simply discussing a point of view or psychological stance. States of mind actually appear to cause changes at the subatomic level. While I do not profess to have even the most rudimentary understanding of quantum mechanics (an admission most physicists also make!), there have been attempts to find an acceptable paradigm for the different phenomena observed in healing practices. Those attempting to explain the non-physical aspects of the healing process have turned to quantum physics due to the absolutely weird and random behavior of particles at the quantum level. Zero Point Energy, based on Heisenberg's Uncertainty Principle, is often invoked to explain paranormal phenomena (including healing).

While this is tempting, one need only observe the repeated phenomena themselves, in the physical world, to know what we should do and not do. The processes may never be fully explained. But we do not have to wait due to the absence of a solid explanation. Experience of the most successful healers points the way.

M.E. Hyland calls attention to the observation that the therapy provider induces change in patients simply by interacting with them.[82] He points out that these phenomena cannot be explained by conventional scientific theories but also cannot be proven adequately by quantum theory, because such tests cannot undergo the usual rigor of testing. As an alternative, Chris Clarke of Southhamptom University[83] claims that quantum "entanglement" is simply the default state of things, at least at the subatomic level. Because of this, certain properties emerge in the living person and these properties make possible non-local (without physical contact) interactions between living systems. Disease is explained by the normal entanglement of quanta (at the subatomic level) becoming disorganized or interrupted. The implication of non-locality is that connections exist that are not limited by space and time.

Hyland asserts that the quantum concept of "emergent entanglement" in physics mirrors Jung's theory of synchronicity, and also the age-old concept of universal mind. In all these, non-local connections are made and manifest themselves.

How this applies to the healing process, according to Hyland, breaks down into four possible explanations. These define the roles of the healer and the patient.

1. The therapist uses some psychological ploy where the patient's psychology is modified in order to activate the healing process.[84]
2. The therapist is an active agent and the patient's energy field is detected and analyzed, and given a corrective directive.
3. The therapist affects the patient because of a non-local connection between them through which

---

82 Hyland, M.E., Emergent Entanglement, Love, and Being, 2004 *Journal of Holistic Healthcare*, 1: 24-29

83 Clarke, C., Entanglement Is Everything, 2004 *Network* 116, 13-16

84 I would point out that conventional medicine does this quite effectively (albeit expensively) with its large institutions, impressive equipment, and widespread advertising.

information is transferred but no energy being transferred (possible due to nonlocal entanglement systems).

4. The therapist does not implant a correctional force but simply observes. His presence allows entanglement to manifest itself. The therapist helps the patient to self-heal by the system re-entangling itself and restoring order, reverting to the default programming.

The thinking reader will recognize that the third and fourth mechanisms are squarely in the quantum entanglement world. It is this fourth mechanism that is the most difficult to arrive at for the average provider of health care (with the exception of psychotherapists, who are taught to adopt the role of observer). But I would suggest that the most appropriate and effective application of Uni-Syn lies in this mechanism.

It is best if the delivery of the purely physical therapies (manipulation, acupuncture, massage, etc.) are coupled with a state of mind in which the therapist and the patient are linked by a created reality: the mental intent of a normalized quantum organization. When the body-mind system is nudged in this direction, it is simply reverting to the normal plan, reassuming what Sheldrake calls a "morphogenetic field".[85]

Returning to the idea of non-local effects, Bell's Incquality Theorem of non-locality seemed to be the conceptual beginning of the idea in science that "everything is connected to everything", although this is a belief that is as old as mankind, and plays a particularly large role in Buddhist thinking.

Studies done in recent decades to establish the power of prayer have yielded interesting results. Directed prayer had significant effects in the trials, but non-directed prayer yielded twice the results. That is, when the participants

[85] Sheldrake, R., *The Presence of the Past,* 2008 HarperCollins pub.

prayed for a specific outcome, they got results that were statistically significant. But when they left it up to a "higher authority" according to their personal beliefs, the outcomes were twice as predictable.[86]

Before we drown in metaphysics let me point out that it has been observed that mental/emotional states don't just take action from brain to brain but interact in some weird way with electronic components. Admit it: Doesn't your computer become even more erratic the more you get mad at it? The creation of this book, for example, was a nightmare of one malfunction after another until I arrived at the mental stance of "I don't care."

Application of Detachment

The first point to make is that having a detached attitude affects not just the therapist's state but the patient's.

There is a complex framework in the human body-mind system composed of neurological structures within connective tissue, the connecting bundles of plexi and resulting reflexes, and their communication with not only the brain within but the electromagnetic field of the body without. **If every aspect of these integrated networks is infused with the consciousness of the individual, then it also creates an antenna grid for outside influences.** When those influences have had negative consequences, it is up to the outside influence of the healer to restore order.

The observational, detached state of that healer seems to create better conditions for the joining of the two psyches for the purpose of solving problems. It is an analogue of the old saying "Two heads are better than one" when illustrating that teamwork is more powerful than isolated problem solving.

---

[86] Dossey, L., *Recovering The Soul, A Scientific and Spiritual Search.* 1997 Bantam, Doubleday, Dell

But this is achieved by stimulating the internal default program of the individual to re-organize, not by imposing a new pattern from the consciousness of the healer.

If you were to arrange a network of fine wires and expose them to an electromagnetic field, there would be measurable current conducted along those wires at a strength far greater than a single wire.

So we are not talking about two completely different realms of reality—the tangible world of nerves, blood vessels, wires and capacitors and the invisible world of spooky immaterial ectoplasms—we are taking about one very long spectrum of reality. To the layman, light, sound, and electricity appear to be completely different entities. But to the scientist, they are all part of a continuum of the electromagnetic spectrum. To someone who understands Uni-Syn, an endocrine gland and a computer chip, a brain and a thought, may not be unrelated.

This leads us back to the concept of the therapist or healer being in an observational state.

For many years, I directed healing thoughts at my patients during treatment, with varying degrees of success. It was only after I had enough "miracle cures" under my belt that I came to expect them. When successful therapy was a "done deal" in my mind and I didn't feel the need to actively direct any kind of healing energy from me to them, I got even better results, much like the prayer experiments. In this case, the "higher power" was the momentum of my past successes and the feeling that I was able to consistently produce results. I didn't have to pray for them; I *knew* they were going to come.

This began to gel for me in a conversation with an extraordinarily successful healer, Dr. Frank Reichlin. "Doctor Frank" was legendary for seeing a hundred-plus patients daily in his prime. I asked him the secret of his success, and he replied, "If there was any 'secret' it was dedication and enthusiasm—the motto was 'Let love radiate, with no expectation of results'."

I would clarify this statement as "Take results for granted and then don't think about them."

Therefore, here are the three conditions that I see as optimal in the healing arts:

(1) Conviction that "Results are guaranteed, so I'm not going to even consider failure".
(2) Non-identification with the healing that takes place: "I'm just the pipeline, not the source."
(3) Loving connection to the patient's world

To again quote Dr. Reichlin, he wrote in a letter:

"Know your true Source and be a conduit for your patients. When you're 'tuned in' everything just flows—but you have to trust that which you're tuned into; the Source, I mean. When *we* are running the show, it's hard work."

In other words, we can, by our best efforts and intentions, produce good work. But it is much more efficient to adopt the right mental stance and allow a higher force[87] to work through us to get the results we desire.

> **"Let love radiate, with no expectation of results."**
>
> **—Frank Reichlin, DC**

And thus we have the fifth principle in Uni-Syn.

[87] It seems to matter little what the higher force is conceived to be. Christians, Buddhists, Jews, Hindus, Muslims, Shintoists and spiritualists all have their prayers answered.

17

REFLEXES: Where Provocation, Polarity and Periodicity Come Together

In the human body, it is the reflexive actions that carry diagnostic and therapeutic information, as we have seen in everything from Chapman's reflexes to Head's Zones, to reactive acupuncture points to tender vertebrae, etc. In Osteopathy, there is a dictum called Feidler's Law, which states that treatment of sensitive areas will affect the disease.[88]

This is not limited to purely manual therapies. Even an oral medicine such as a homeopathic remedy functions by way of such reflexes. If the administration of the medicine is the *provocation*, and the homeopathic indications respect *polarity* (action of the remedy provoking an opposite response from the body), then the dose duration and the rest/development phase of the reactions is the *periodicity*.

The response to a homeopathic medicine is clearly an activation of a reflex phenomenon (the body reverses the disease process due to the similarity of the remedy characteristics). In the same way, we instinctively press a tender spot on the body. This seems to be counter-intuitive, since it is already painful and continued and forceful pressure would surely aggravate the pain. Yet, creating pain

[88] Also, that treatments applied to sensitive areas nearest to the spine are more effective than at more distant points.

that *mimics* the injurious force that caused the pain tends to relieve it—what could be called a manual homeopathic effect.

This instinct is likely what gave birth to massage therapy millennia ago, but it is further expressed in Japanese acupuncture, where the needling is generally much less vigorous and of less duration than Chinese acupuncture. The aforementioned Dr. John Amaro, who combines chiropractic manipulation and acupuncture in his clinic, uses short-duration laser stimulation of the points extensively and has insisted that "less is more" (expressing the fourth principle of *minimization*). Bowen Therapy uses very brief soft tissue moves to activate these reflexes, achieving minimization as well as the other "Three Ps".

The main locations for such point stimulations (*provocations*) as we have seen, are nearly identical for the various systems we have reviewed. What remains to be shown is a cohesive routine that synthesizes the many disciplines so that any type of practitioner will have at hand a comprehensive treatment that is at the same time simple and efficient. Doctors of Naprapathy should in particular find this easy to incorporate into their fascia-based practice, and massage therapists will find that they can do more for their clients in less time.

Thus, the Uni-Syn General Treatment as presented here stands as a go-to routine for balancing a patient as well as a health maintenance method. It is curious how electrical readings of the acupuncture meridians change dramatically after one of these sessions. Those readers who perform point measurement or meridian analysis are encouraged to do before-and-after studies.

In the protocols outlined here, the various provocation points to be stimulated can be treated with the fingers, knuckles, or a manual therapy tool such as a "T bar", Graston tool or gua sha implement. It need not contact bare skin, as long as the maneuver stretches the skin and fascia during the movement in order to create a piezoelectric response in the tissues. The author demonstrates a Bowen Therapy-style manual provocation in these illustrations, where the connective tissue is moved to an end point, then while continuing to apply pressure, the tissues are flicked back in the opposite direction.

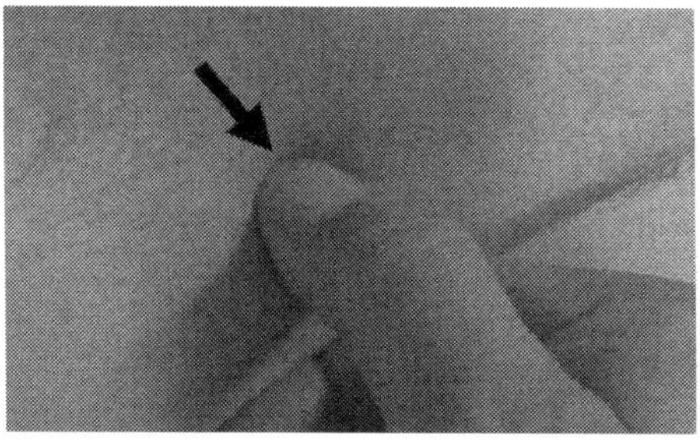

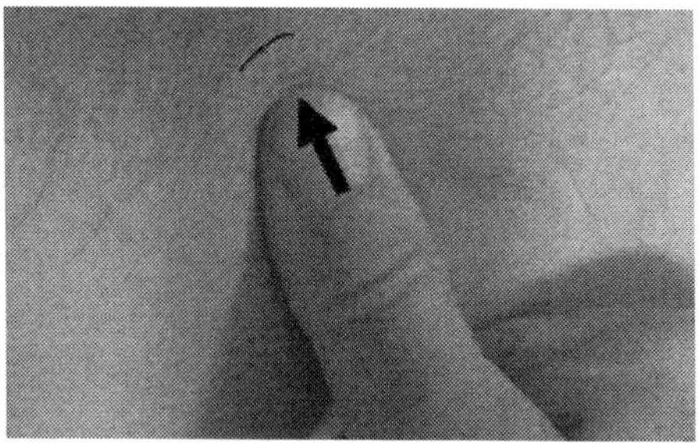

This is a method long used in Shiatsu in Japan, but later established by Australian Tom Bowen to arouse the healing reaction. Dr. Leo Sears, founder of the Sears Chiropractic Sanitarium in Denver, Colorado, made use of the exact same movements that he called “”nerve goading”. But any type of stimulation that creates a piezoelectric response (certainly including piezoelectricity itself) will have a similar effect. Therefore, any type of practitioner can make use of these protocols, mixing and matching as needed.

Follow the Uni-Syn principles that have been expounded upon here, including the practice of treating the unaffected side first. When the problem being treated is one-sided, the choice is clear, but in a bilateral presentation, treat the less affected side first.

The other contribution Tom Bowen made with his Bowen Therapy is the practice of pausing and leaving the room at various points during the treatment, something unique among therapeutic systems and the value of which has already been discussed in the chapter on Periodicity. It is beyond question that this is a crucial element in the efficacy of these methods, and those following these protocols should not fail to include it.

GENERAL UNI-SYN TREATMENT

This is a suggested procedure for routine use. It follows somewhat the pattern of the Collins Universal Naturopathic Tonic Treatment already described in Chapter Eight. It can be used to stimulate a healing response no matter what the disorder, with extra attention and stimulation in additional specific areas as needed.

Step One is performed manually. The subject lies in the prone position. The operator stands at the head of the treatment table and begins with the thumbs each over the T1-T2 junction with the tips of the thumbs almost touching under the T1 spinous process.

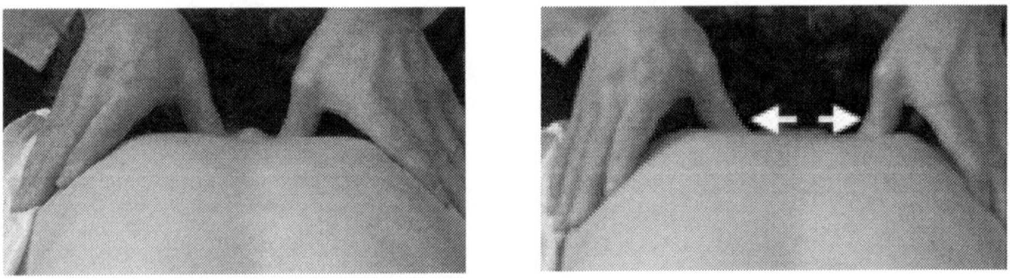

Step One

Pressing down, the thumbs are dragged toward the midline and then drawn apart laterally to stretch the skin and fascia and roll it over the prominence of the Longissimus muscle, which can be felt beneath the more superficial Trapezius. This stimulates both the vertebral points and associated points at that spinal level. Draw the thumbs apart as far as a hand width lateral to the midline, leaving them pressing on the lateral channel of the bladder meridian, as can be seen in the illustration.

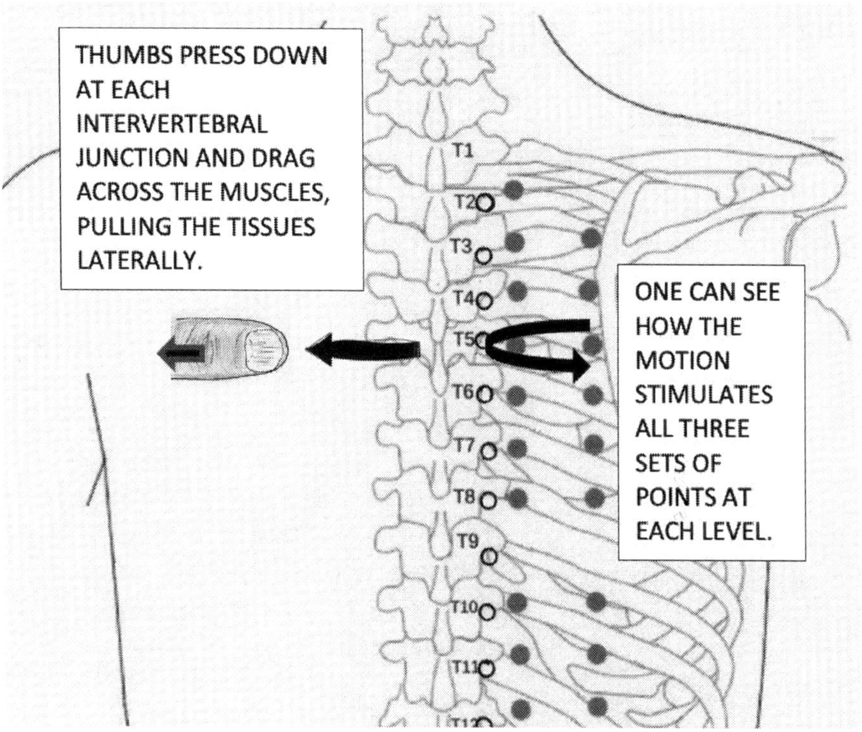

THUMBS PRESS DOWN AT EACH INTERVERTEBRAL JUNCTION AND DRAG ACROSS THE MUSCLES, PULLING THE TISSUES LATERALLY.
ONE CAN SEE HOW THE MOTION STIMULATES ALL THREE SETS OF POINTS AT EACH LEVEL.
T1
T2
T3
T4
T5
T6
T7
T8
T9
T10
T11

In this way, all three sets of points at each spinal level is stimulated. If a tool is used, one side may be done at a time.

Releasing contact, place the thumbs or tool at the T2-T3 junction and perform the same maneuver. Repeat for each spinal level, moving caudally. Typically when one reaches the T6 level or so, the clinician is bending forward too far to be efficient, so reposition yourself at the side of the table facing the cephalic direction, and continue the maneuver down the spine until completing the L5-S1 junction.

Step Two

From your position on the left side of the table, curl the fingers of the right hand under the subject's right anterior superior iliac crest. It helps to insert a folded towel against the body to prevent tickling.

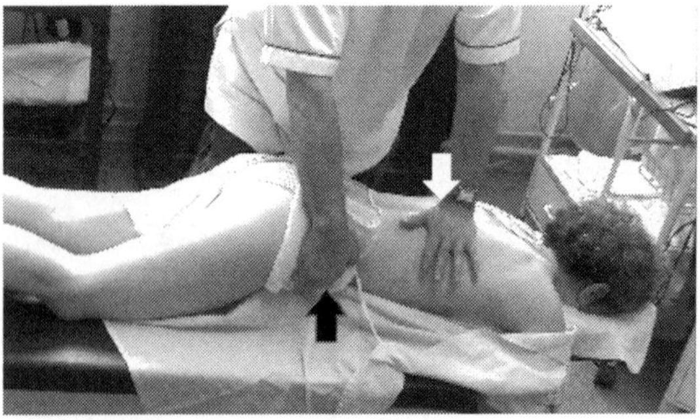

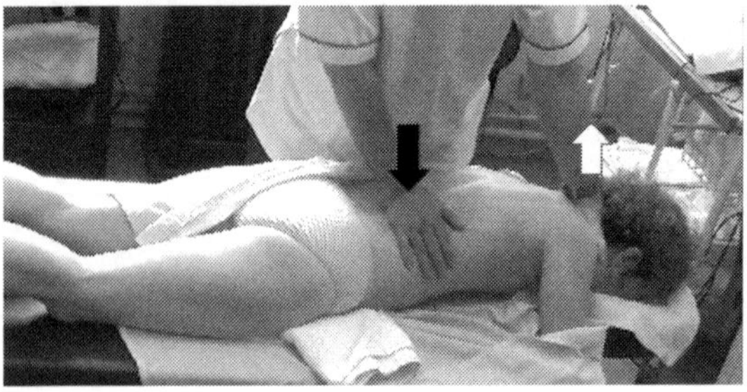

1. Place the left hand on the subject's right scapula. While pressing down with the left hand, pull up on the hip with the right hand to create torsion in the spine and rib cage. Hold for two seconds and release.
2. Next hook your left hand under subject's left shoulder, press down on the subject's right hip with the right hand, and twist the torso in this direction.

3. Change your position to the right side of the table. Curl the fingers of your left hand under the subject's left anterior superior iliac crest, using a towel as before. This will be the mirror image of Step Two. Place the right hand on the subject's left scapula. While pressing down with the right, pull up on the hip with the left hand to create torsion in the spine and rib cage once again. Hold for two seconds and release. Next hook your right hand under subject's right shoulder, press down on the subject's left hip with the left hand, and twist the torso as you did on the opposite side.

Step Three

Make drawing movements with the thumb (or tool) across the left side of the sacrum, diagonally at the level of S2 and again at S4. Then dig with a knuckle, thumb, or tool into the "dimple point" of the Gluteus (acupuncture point GB-30), using a rotary motion until a response is given by the subject (vocal or muscle twitch). Repeat same procedure on the right side of the sacrum.

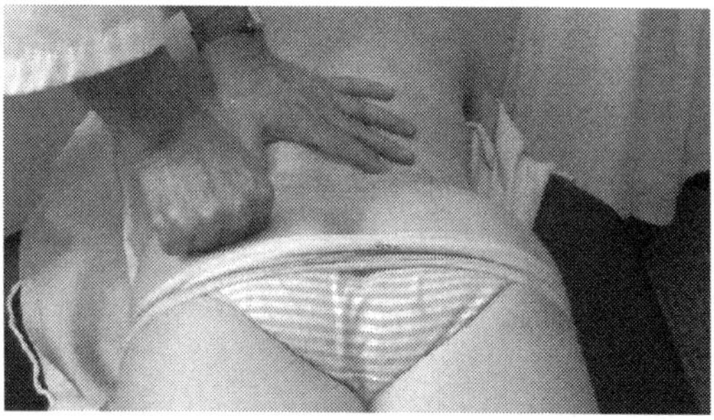

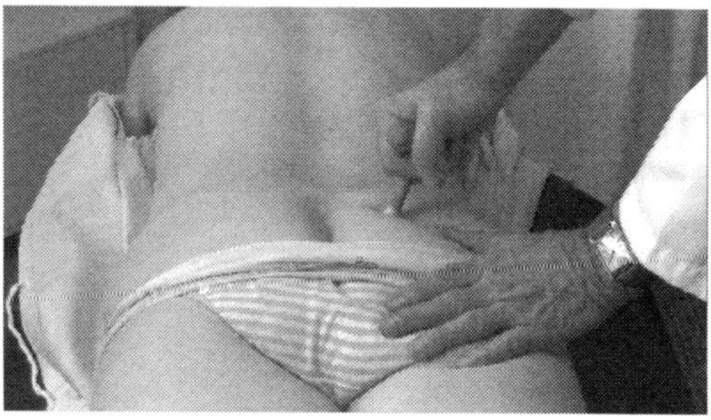

Step Four

Set a timer for two minutes and leave the room, instructing the subject to remain motionless.

Step Five

Returning to the subject, place yourself again at the head of the table, facing caudally. Press on the left Trapezius just lateral to T1 and draw the thumb or tool diagonally across the muscle to elicit the reaction. Reposition the thumb laterally and repeat. Move position laterally once more and create the reaction a final time, posterior to the acromio-clavicular junction. Now repeat the same sequence on the subject's right side.

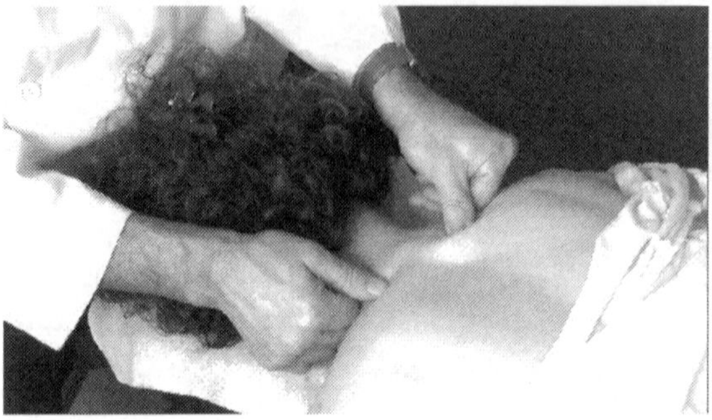

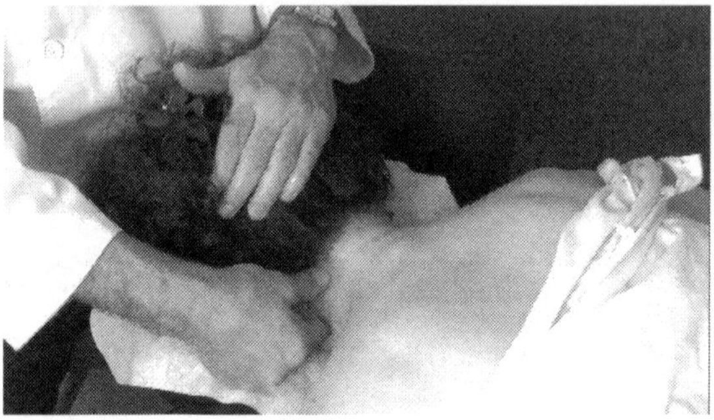

Step Six

1. Press toward the midline and then draw the right thumb across the subject's left suboccipital region, laterally to stretch the tissues and elicit the response.
2. Then press and draw the left thumb across the subject's right side. You should feel yourself rolling over directly the upper Trapezius and the Splenius Capitas at the base of the skull, provoking points UB-10 and GB-20 (illustrated later).

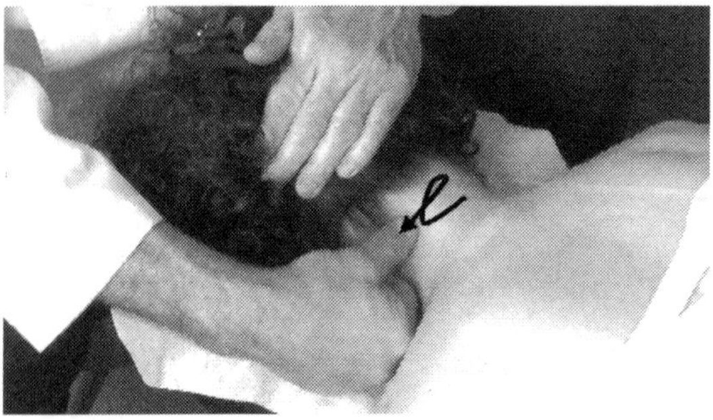

Step Seven

1. Place the right thumb on the posterior neck at the level of the left C3 transverse process, and make a rotary movement followed by a lateral pull.
2. Follow with the mirror image on the left side. You should feel the muscle rebound.

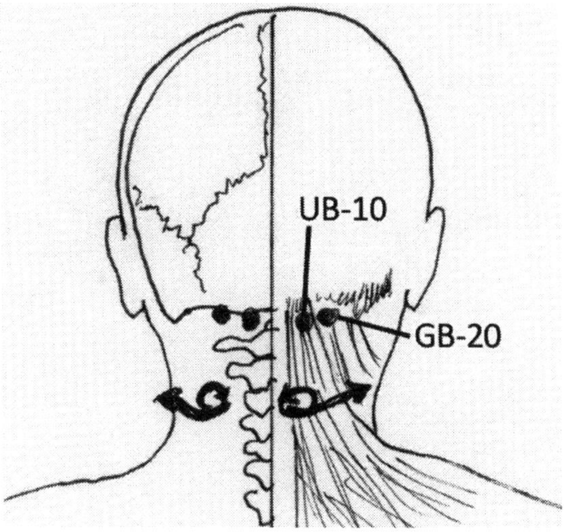

Points used in Steps Six and Seven

Step Eight

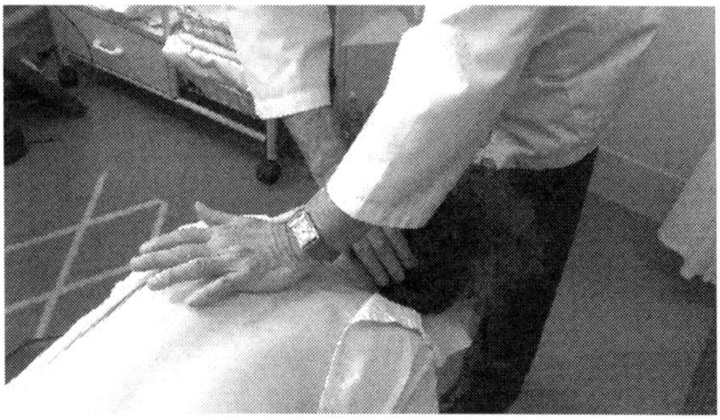

1. Still standing at the head of the table, ask the subject to turn the head to the subject's left. Pressing down with the right hand to stabilize the head, cross arms pressing with the left palm against the area lateral to T1 to T3, on subject's left. Stretch the paracervical muscles.
2. Then ask the subject to turn the head the other way, and perform the mirror image.

Step Nine

Ask the subject to turn over in the supine position and rest there. Return in two minutes.

Step Ten

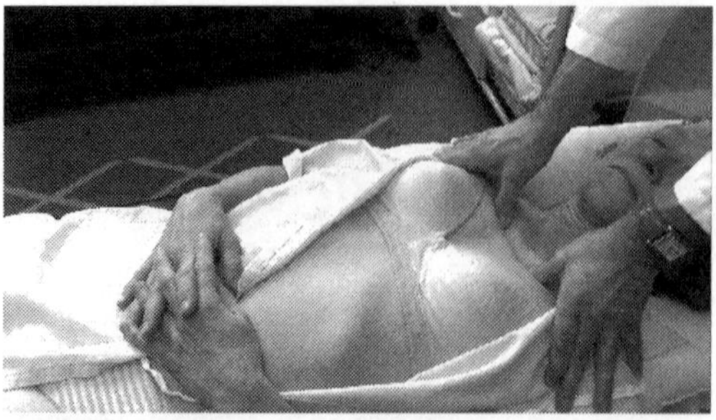

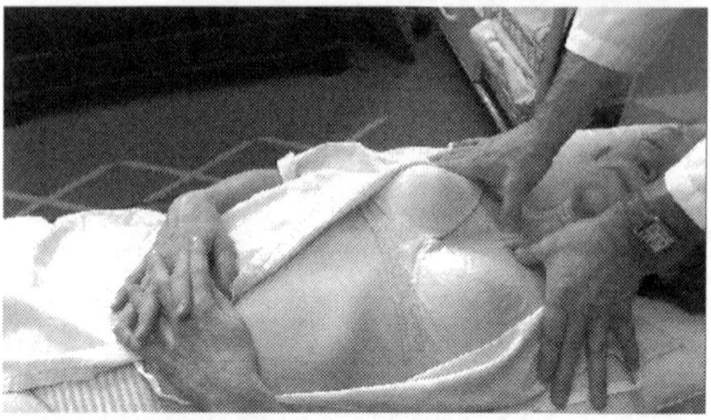

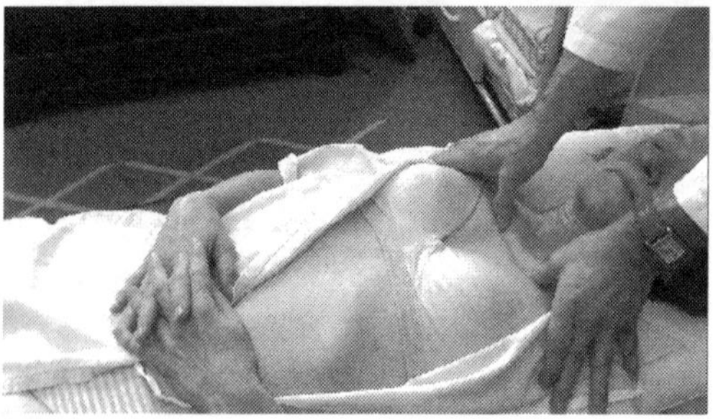

1.Make drawing movements with the thumbs laterally in several short bursts along the depression under the clavicle, beginning at the manubrium and ending at the acromion. Treat both sides.

2.Now move inferiorly and place the thumbs in the first intercostal space against the manubrium. Press and slide over the border of the manubrium medially, then reverse direction and draw the thumbs laterally. This is the same movement as in Step One, along the spine. Repeat this move for each intercostal space, dragging the tissues slightly over the sternum and then laterally. Cease after the sixth intercostal space has been treated[89]. It may be judicious, if the subject is female, to take the subject's own fingers and use them to make the contacts. The effect is not diminished if the clinician guides the fingers to make the unique flipping motion that results in the piezoelectric response in the fascia.

[89] This follows the path of Chapman's neurolymphatic points as already illustrated, but also that of the kidney meridian, which Amaro postulates is an extension of the line of the vertebral points on the posterior.

Step Eleven

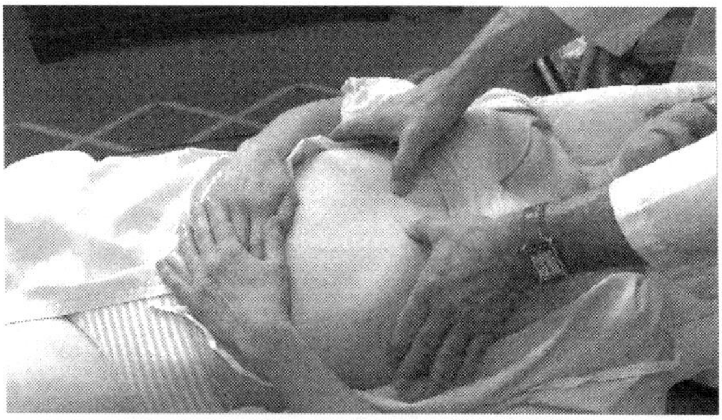

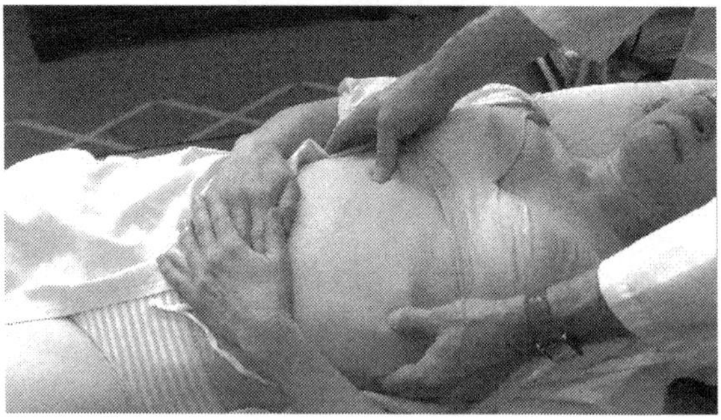

1. Curl the fingertips just under the ribs close to the xiphoid process and slide them laterally to create the now familiar dragging/flipping motion to elicit the reaction from the reflex. On terminating the motion, the fingers should have "flipped" over to the anterior surface. Move laterally and repeat. Repeat until the entire surface of the costal cartilage has been stimulated.

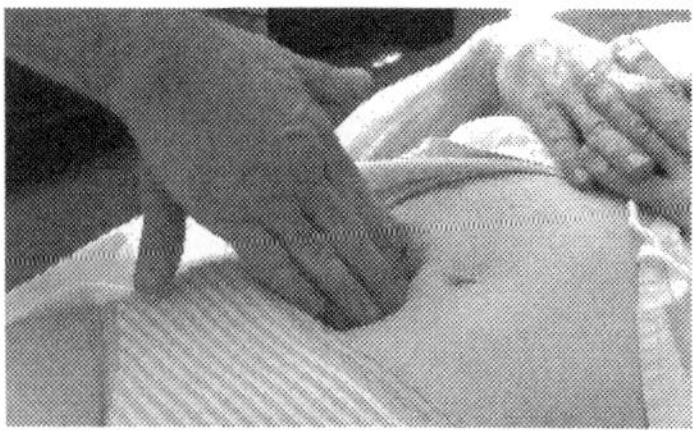

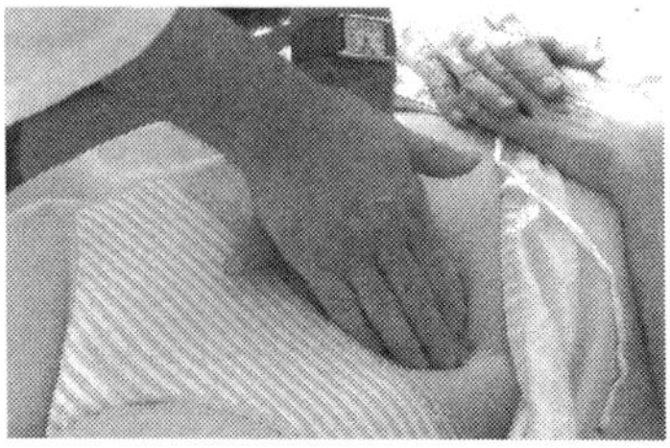

2. Make circular kneading motions across the abdomen, proceeding from the right lower quadrant, following the path of the ascending colon, transverse colon, and descending colon to arrive at the left lower quadrant. To relieve the "tickle factor", the clinician can use the subject's fingers for contact as before. There is no attempt in this case to stretch and rebound the fascia. Simply knead firmly and gently in a circle.

Step Twelve

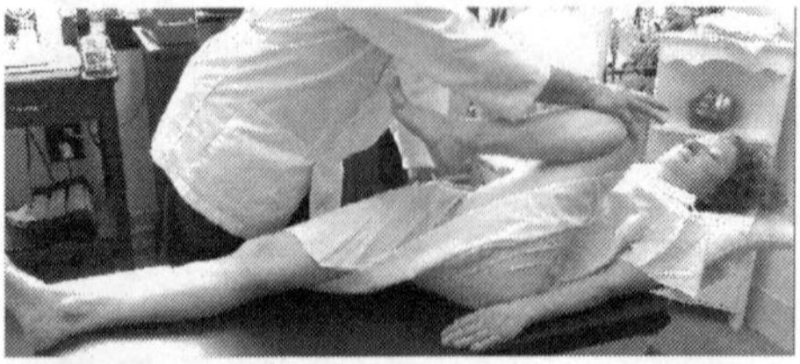

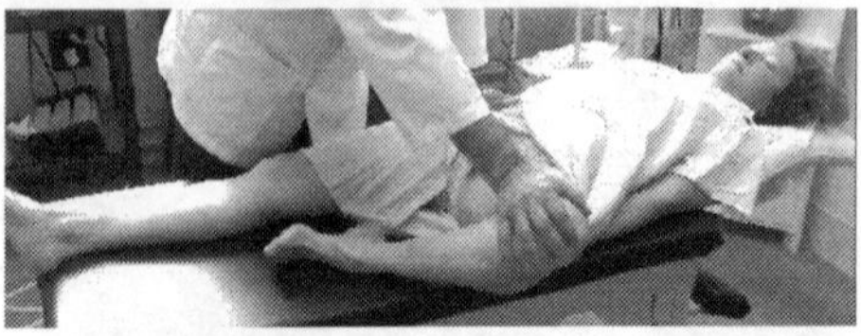

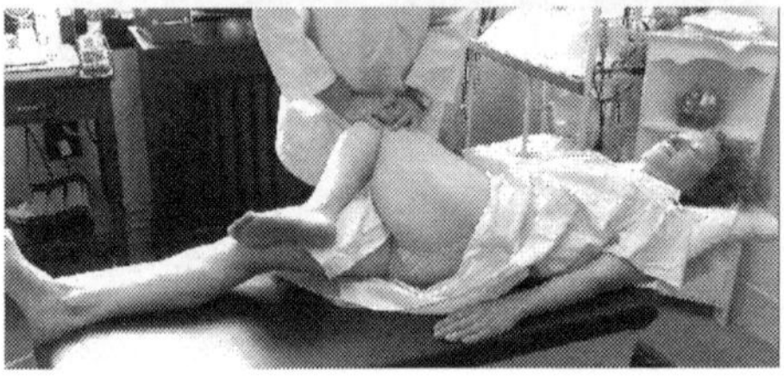

1.Ask subject to breathe in and out. On the exhalation, flex the left leg so that the thigh touches the abdomen.
2.From there, abduct the leg (with the knee at 90 degrees flexion) while using the other hand to stabilize the opposite iliac crest. Stretch as far as is comfortable for the subject.
3.Now reverse direction and draw the leg across the abdomen in adduction, using the closest hand to stabilize the shoulder on that side to prevent the subject from rolling. Again, stretch to tolerance for a few seconds.
4. Repeat sequence on opposite side.

Step Thirteen

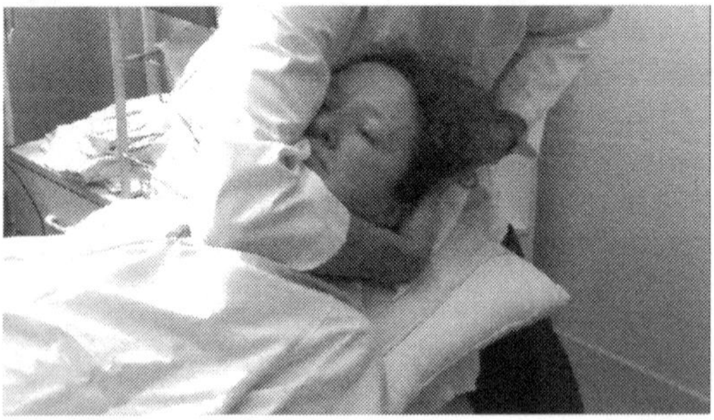

Return to the head of the table. Encircle the subject's head with your dominant arm, with subject's chin nestled in the crook of your elbow. Stabilize the head with the other hand placed firmly on the forehead. Say you are going to stretch the spine and to tell you when subject feels the stretch. Holding the head firmly, lean back slowly to increase the longitudinal stretch and stop when subject indicates feeling the stretching action. At that moment, very briefly flex the biceps of the arm encircling the jaw of the subject. The momentary crowding under the chin will create an impulse that creates an extremely brief and mild traction on the atlanto-occipital joint.

Step Fourteen

Using the fingernail, fore-knuckle, or other implement against the scalp, stimulate in a brisk, circular motion the acupuncture point GV-20 at the apex of the cranium. This is done no more than seven rotations and then stopped.

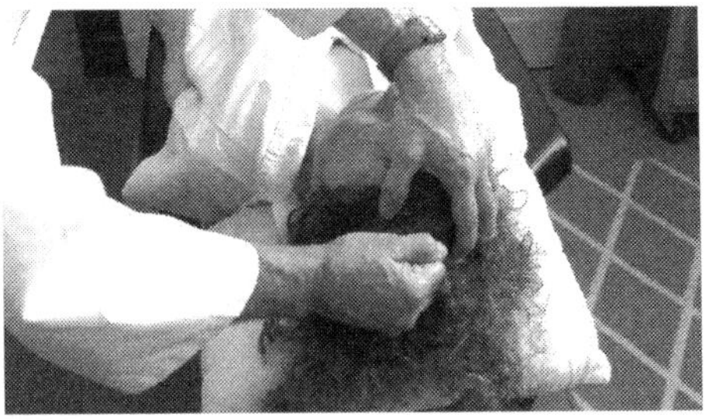

GV-20 is located on the midline where it is crossed by an imaginary line connecting the apex of each ear.

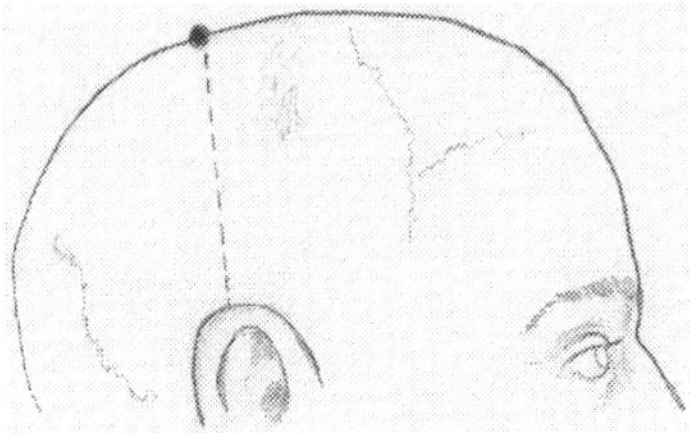

Step Fifteen

Subject is left to rest for two minutes before being allowed to rise.

Stimulation can be manual (as described in the General Uni-Syn Treatment), or instrument-assisted (T-bar, spring-loaded activator, etc.), or electrical (piezo electrical stimulator, etc.). The main criterion is that the provocation creates a momentary sensation that jolts the fascia into producing a piezoelectric response).

These protocols are excellent for the practitioner who uses manual therapies, such as a massage therapist. They are equally good, however, as a guide for an acupuncture practitioner, or a chiropractor who wishes to add to, or substitute for, joint manipulation. Naturopathic practitioners run the gamut as to what therapies they may use, but these maneuvers are applicable for any type of practitioner.

These procedures draw equally from both the long-used Chapman neurolymphatic reflexes and the more modern Bowen Therapy. However, both these methods are unintentionally performing non-needle acupuncture, because the reflexes are largely the same. So I have used well-known acupuncture points as landmarks in many cases to both emphasize the oneness of these methods and to better illustrate the procedures.

For example, if we look at the Bowen protocol for upper respiratory problems, we see a "move" (as it is termed in Bowen Therapy) being made along the clavicle. Chiropractors will notice that the Chapman point for the nasal reflex is in the vicinity, in the first rib space, which also corresponds to the acupuncture Kidney point 27, instantly recognizable to acupuncturists. The Bowen move along the mandible and the last posterior neck move seem to collectively activate the posterior Chapman nasal reflex, which is described by Owens[90] thusly:

---

[90] Owens, Charles; An Endocrine Interpretation of Chapman's Reflexes, Academy for Applied Osteopathy; 2nd ed. (1963)

Placing the finger under the angle of the jaw, as if you were going to draw a line across the face to parallel the line of the mouth and shoving the finger backward until you come in line with the transverse process of the vertebra, you will find an excessively sensitive gangliform contraction the size of a half pea.

By thorough relaxation of this contraction you will be able to give a sense of complete clearing of the nasal passages in rhinitis or hay-fever.

These procedures have proven their worth in my clinic for many years and their hybrid nature (from multiple sources) makes it the most expedient to simply call them "Uni-Syn" protocols.

Low Back Dysfunction:

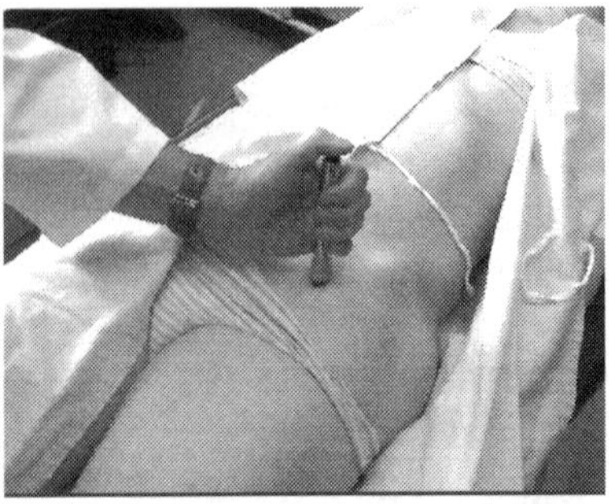

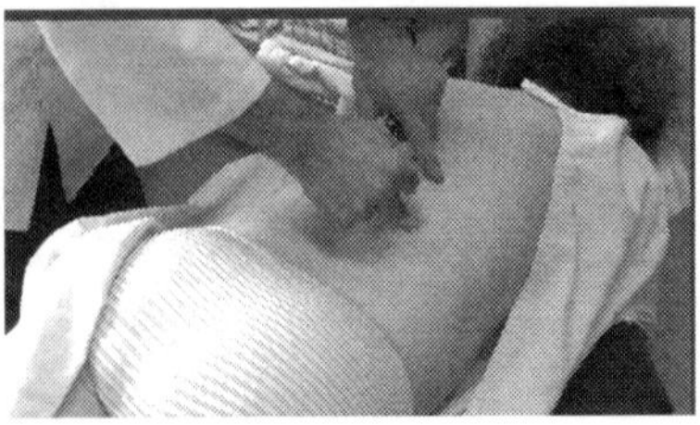

1.Subject lying supine. Stimulate point St-30 on the anterior of the hip in the fold formed when the hip is flexed. It lies on the mammary line. With the legs extended, stimulate this point on both sides, then have subject turn over to prone position.

2.Subject prone. Stimulate the vertebral points at the lower borders of the spinous processes of T11 and UB-20, an inch or so lateral. This lies over the kidneys and represents what the founder of Chiropractic called K.P., or "kidney place". Acupuncturists will recognize this as being at the level of GV-6, and is the associated point for the spleen. A tool is being used in the illustration.

3. Stimulate the vertebral points and UB-23 (not illuistrated) bilaterally, at the level of L2-L3 (same movement as in Uni-Syn General Treatment, pressing toward the midline and dragging laterally).

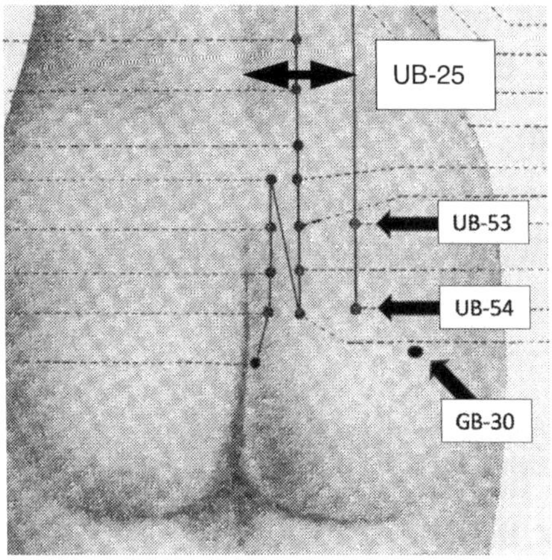

4. Stimulate the vertebral points and UB-25 bilaterally, at the level of L4-L5 (same movement as in Uni-Syn General Treatment, pressing toward the midline and dragging laterally).
5. Stimulate UB-53 and UB-54 one one side, then the other. They are located 3 units lateral to the border of the sacrum at the level of S2 and S4 respectively, and the tissues can be stretched over the sacrum and then rolled back to create the stimulation. Then stimulate GB-30 in the Gluteal dimple with a circular motion, bilaterally.

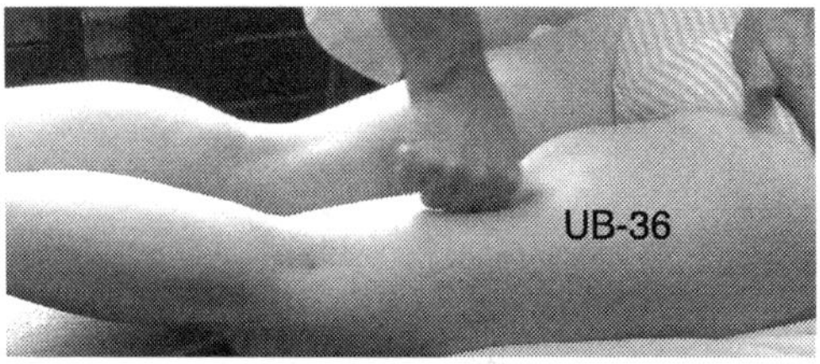

6. Stimulate UB-36 on one leg with a circular motion, then GB-33, and GB-31 with a dragging motion posteriorly. Repeat for the other leg.

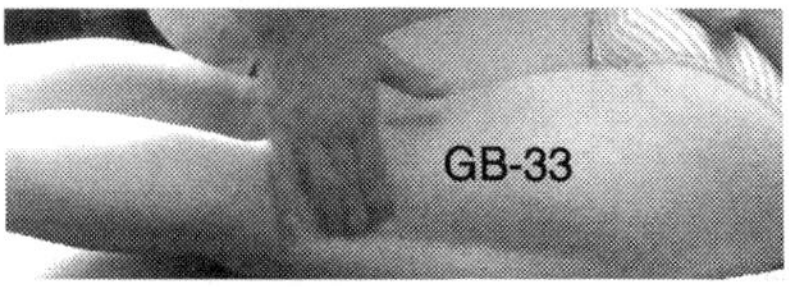

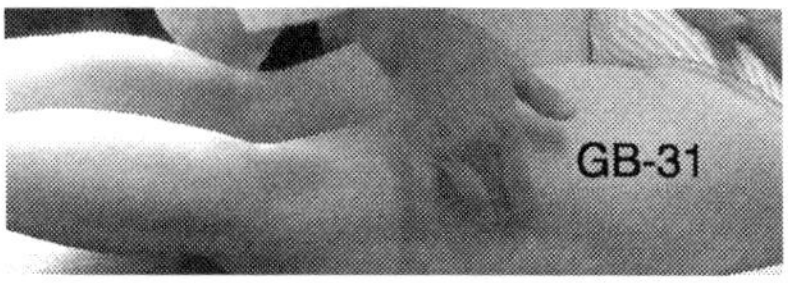

7. Require subject to rest for two minutes before rising. Adjunct therapies such as hot pack, infrared, or short wave may be applied after this time. Do not use mechanical vibration or any other stimulation immediately after the point stimulation.

1. **Upper Back Dysfunction:**
Patient in supine position. Stimulate the neurolymphatic reflexes and kidney meridian points starting from the depression between the first rib and the inferior border of the clavicle, moving laterally to KI-27. Do this bilaterally. Reposition the hands in the next rib space and stimulate the next set of points. Continue until you reach the mammary line or 5th rib space.

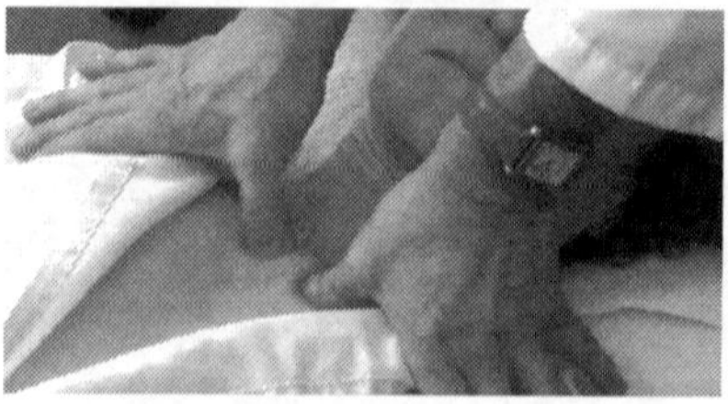

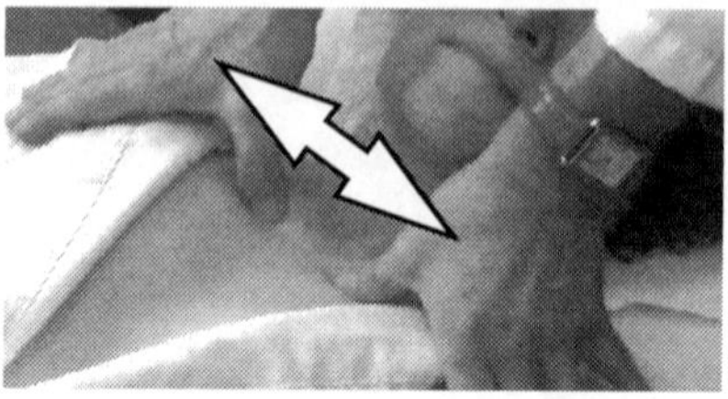

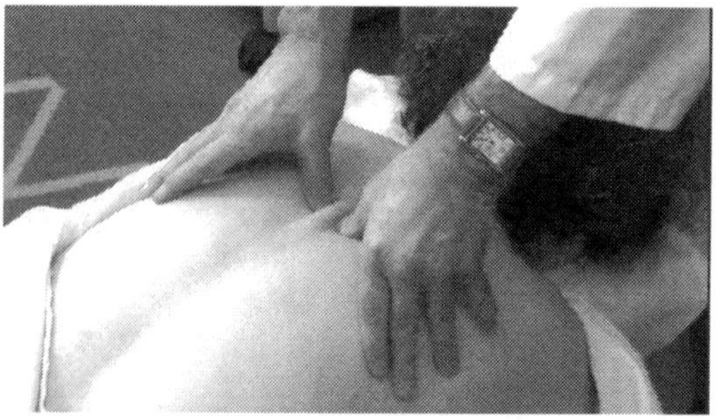

2.Have the subject turn over to prone posture and rest for 2 minutes before proceeding.

3.Subject in prone position, stimulate the vertebral points at T5-T6, moving laterally to include UB-15, bilaterally. This area was referred to by the founder of Chiropractic as C.P., or "center place". Reposition yourself in a caudal direction and stimulate the next set of points at the T6-T7 level. Acupuncturists will recognize these two sets of points as the associated points for the heart and diaphragm.

4. Stimulate SI-9, about one unit superior to the posterior axillary fold. The tissue is very pliable in this region, so manual stimulation will necessitate stretching and rolling the fascia against the Latissimus. Draw the tissues toward the arm, then reverse direction and drag it diagonally on a line pointing toward T3. Treat both sides.

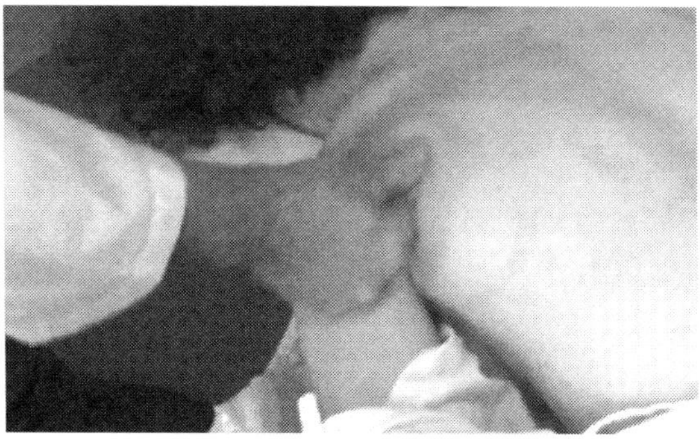

5. Stimulate SI-15, a point 2 units lateral to the inferior border of the spinous process of C7. Provoke the tissues medially[91]. Depending on the subject's body, you may have to make the provocation inferiorly or superiorly over the Trapezius. Repeat on other side.

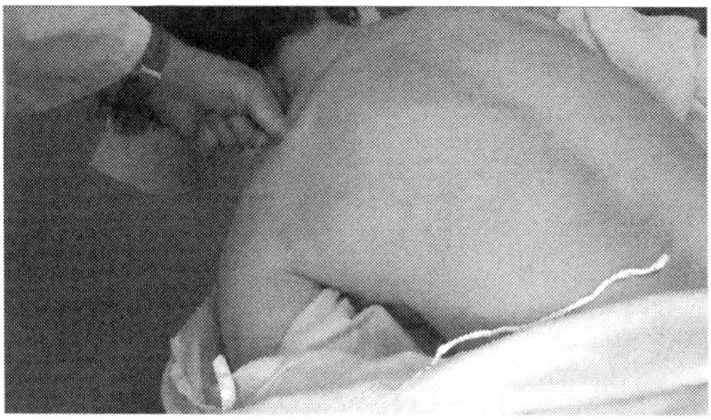

6. Allow subject to rest 2 minutes before continuing or rising.

[91] This not only has upper back, neck, shoulder, and respiratory effects, it also stimulates Voll point VUB-10c (stellate ganglion) and the classical point UB-11 (action on the osseous system). See page 187 for illustration.

Neck Dysfunction:

1. Subject lies supine. Palpate the anterior shoulder, inferior to the glenohumeral joint and medial to the bicipital tendon sheath. There is a point inferior to the insertion of the Subscapularis tendon that can be exquisitely tender when the neck is dysfunctional[92]. Treat this point bilaterally with medium pressure in circular motions, or with a device if you are using one.

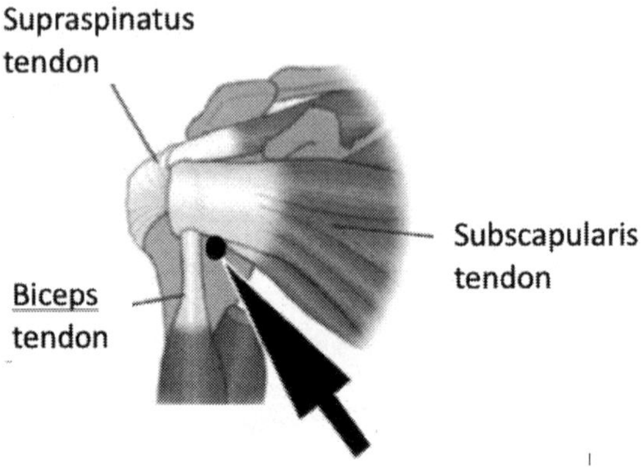

Several points in the upper back and neck areas will be provoked in the following sequences. The large number of such points in the region, with their local and distal effects on the body, can be seen on the chart on the next page. The neurological and visceral connections to these points were established by extensive research in Germany and were not intended for any kind of bodywork. Still, their effects are elicited by the provocation method of stretching the fascia and dragging it in an opposite direction to create the piezoelectric response.

Once one has mastered locating the points used in this Uni-Syn protocol, one can proceed to these points while having the subject remain supine, provoking them with an underhanded contact. However, it is helpful in the beginning to practice with the subject prone. We will illustrate it in this way.

[92] Due to decreased lymphatic fluid draining from the paracervical muscles.

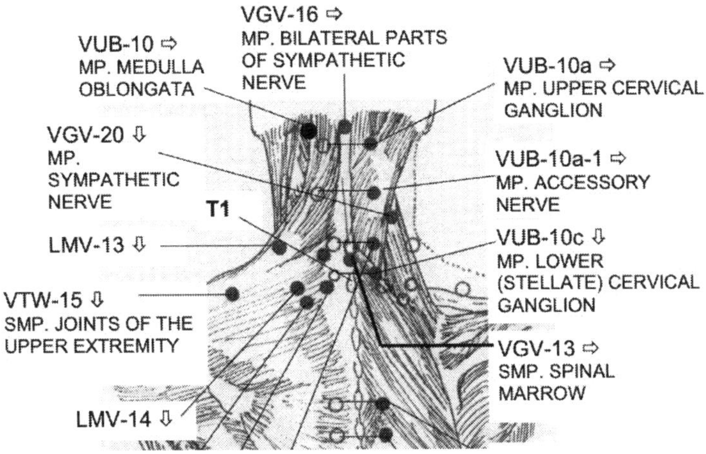

The many points in the region.

2. With the subject in the prone position for clarity, roll the thumb over the Trapezius and contact SI-15, lateral to the C7 spinous process bilaterally. Press the fingers in a caudal direction, dragging the tissues with them, then reverse direction, drawing them to the superior border of the Trapezius and allowing the fascia to spring. Move the fingers to a new position laterally and repeat, until you reach the acromion.

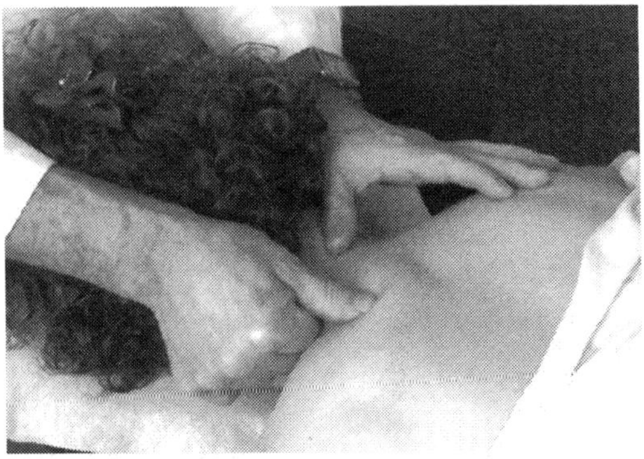

3. Place the fingers under the occiput and drag laterally, one side and then the other. Spring the large tendons to create the reflex. This stimulates Voll point

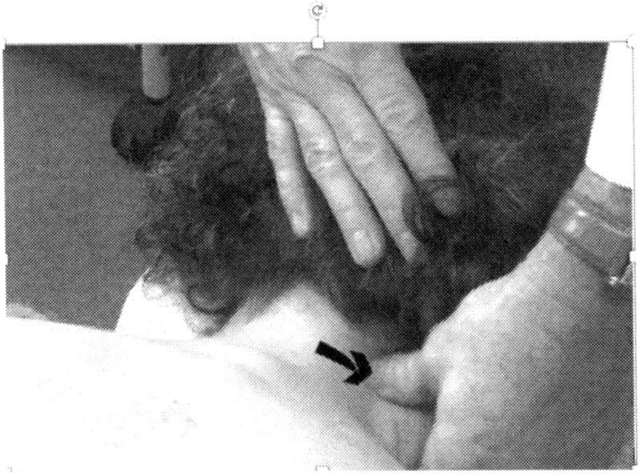

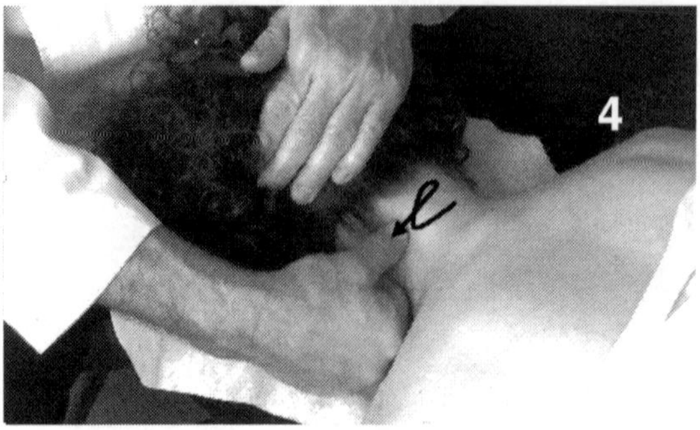

VUB-10a (upper cervical ganglion).

4. Move one finger to the level of C3, stretch the tissues and trace a circle quickly with the pad of the finger, terminating with a move laterally. Break contact and repeat on the other side. This stimulates Voll point VUB-10a (accessory nerve).
5. Allow subject to rest for 2 minutes before moving.

TMJ Dysfunction

(First perform **neck dysfunction** protocol.)

1. In supine position, have subject place a knuckle between the front teeth to maintain an open temperomandibular joint during the procedure. Tell subject to not bite down on finger.
2. Palpate the condyle and press with the pad of the finger, or a padded tool. Drawing the tissues anteriorly, reverse direction toward the ear, creating a "flipping" sensation over the condyle. This causes a provocation of points St-7 and GB-2.

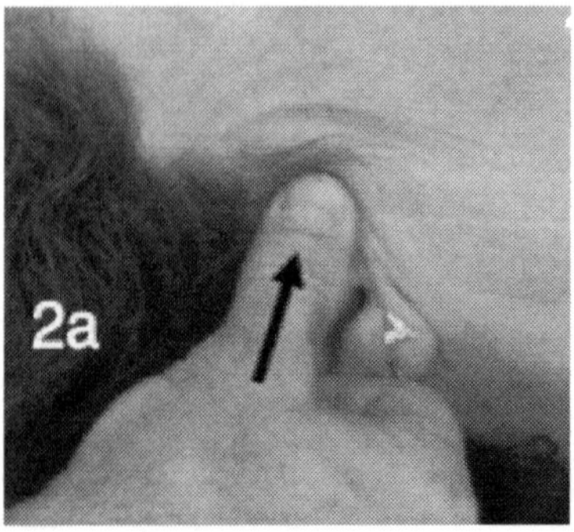

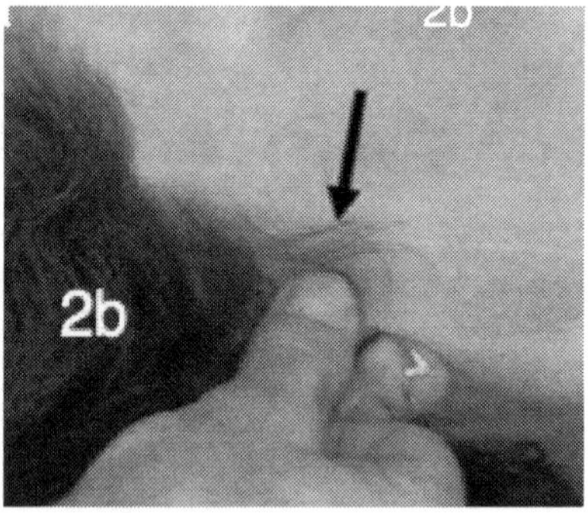

3. Perform a similar movement in another plane by drawing the tissues in a cephalic direction over the condyle, then reversing to move caudally. The subject will usually react to this provocation.
4. Palpate the ramus of the mandible. Draw the tissues toward the earlobe, then reverse direction quickly toward the border of the mandible at midpoint.
5. Palpate the anterior border of the Auricularis superior and make a firm pressure, drawing the tissues anteriorly toward the Auricularis anterior, then reversing to create a provocation.

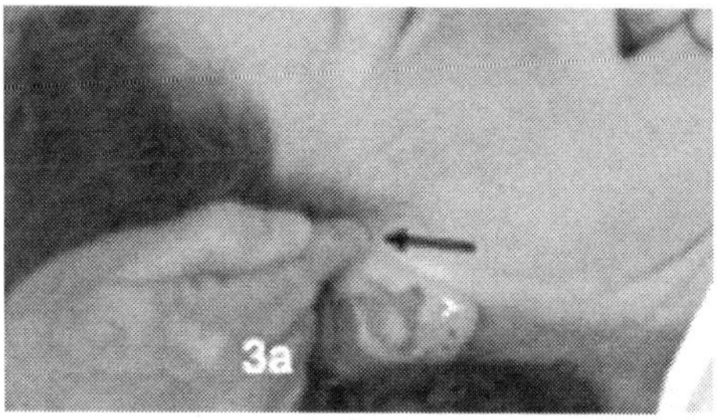

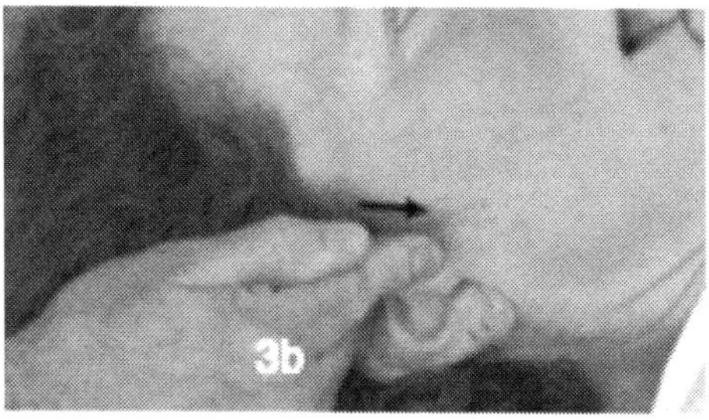

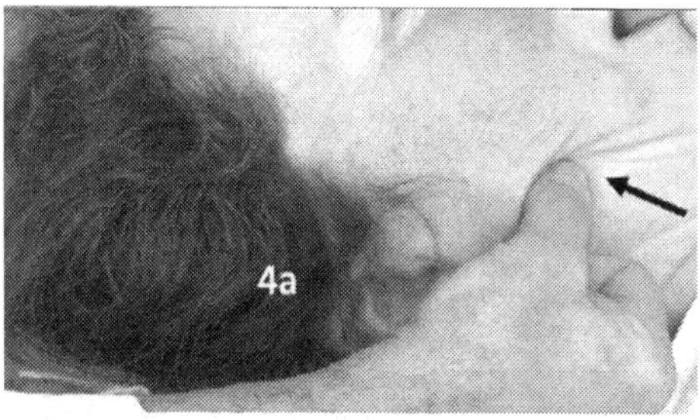

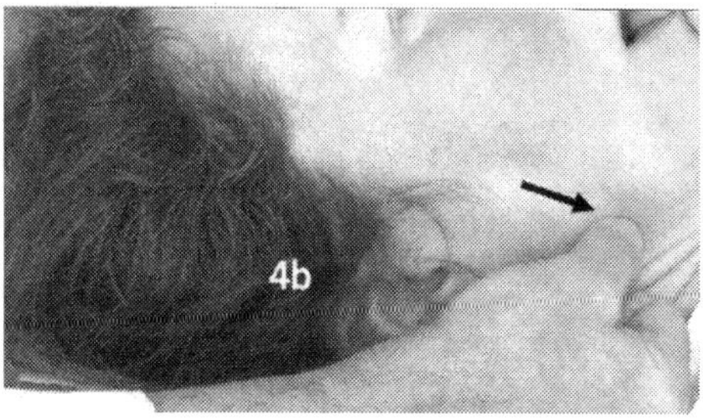

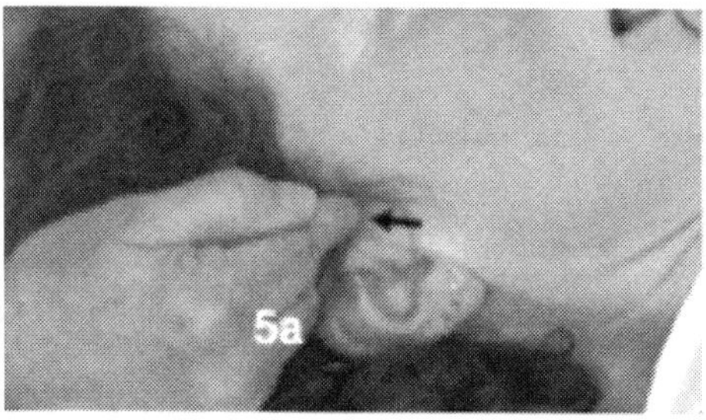

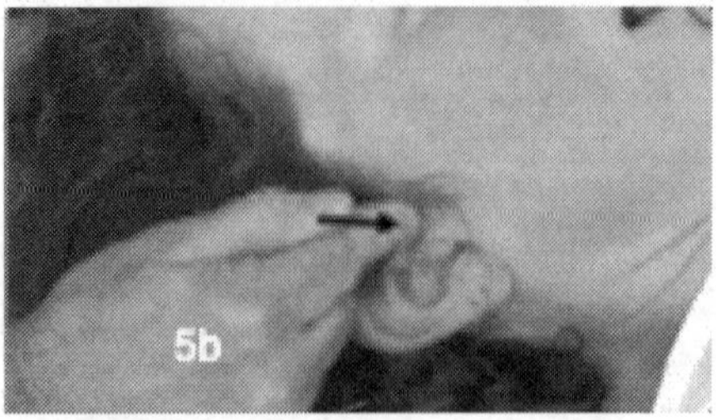

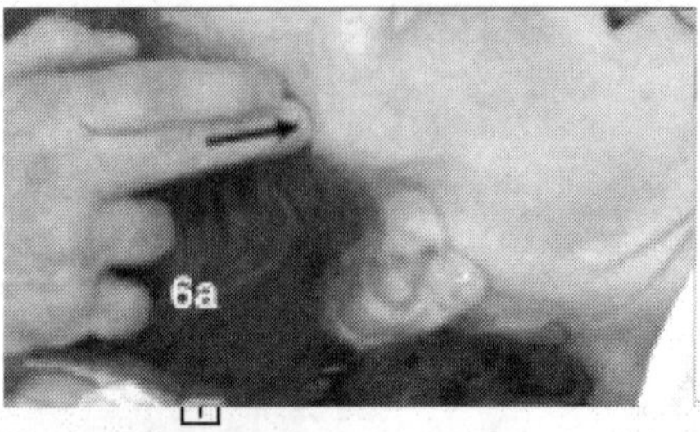

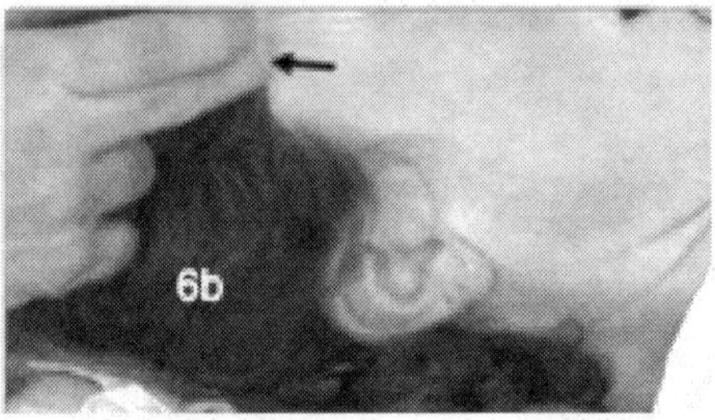

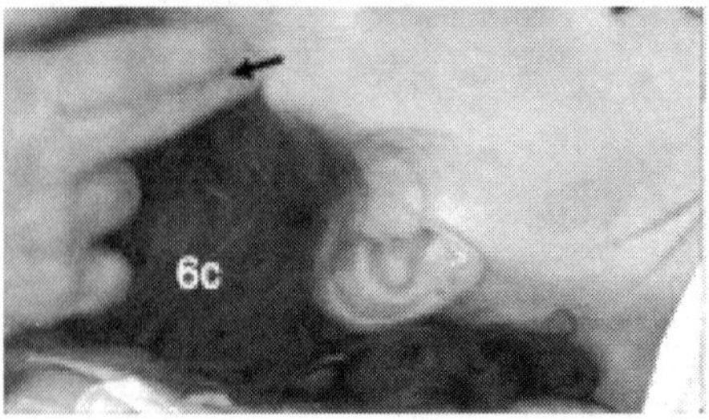

6.Make a series of provocations following the Sphenoid bone at its junction with the Parietal, springing the tissues posteriorly over onto the Parietal. It helps to aim the movement toward the vertex.

7.Perform entire sequence on other side.

8.Provoke the point TW-3 on the dorsum of the hand bilaterally. Press on the point and drag the tissues proximally. TW-3 is a distal reflex point for any problem in the temporo-mandibular joint, and well known to acupuncturists. It is a simple matter to elicit the provocation with a tool or with the fingertip, as stimulating the spot will typically cause an electrical sensation or a deep ache in the hand.

To those familiar with Bowen Therapy, I have added the last provocations to the usual protocol as I have found that they produce better results. Chronic tension in the Temporalis muscle is typically present in TMJ syndrome.

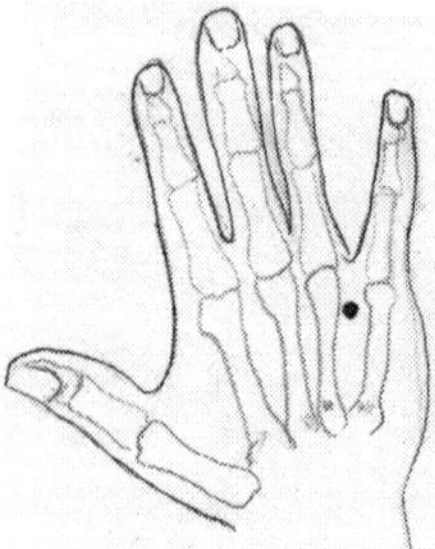
TW-3

Shoulder Dysfunction

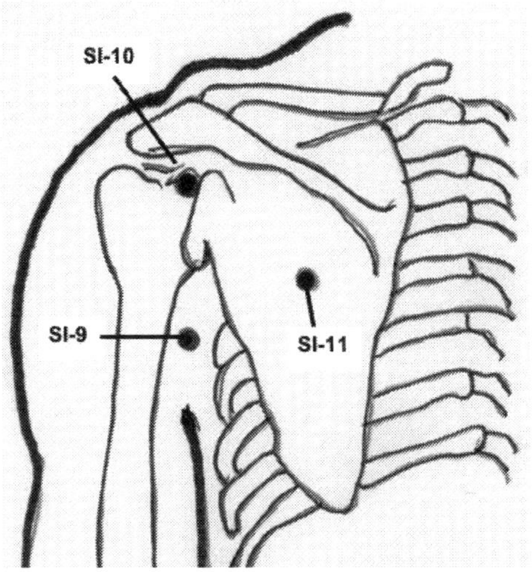

Treat, as always, the unaffected or less affected shoulder first.
The sequence may be done twice if needed in a single session, but do not repeat for seven days.

1. Locate point SI-9 approximately one inch superior to the end of the posterior axillary fold. Press deeply and roll the tissue diagonally in a cephalic direction, terminating at point SI-11 as seen in the illustration.
2. Press deeply on SI-11. It is located in the center of the infrascapular fossa so you will feel a depression under the tissues. Without releasing the pressure on the point, drag the tissues diagonally toward the acromion and point SI-10, allowing them to spring back, creating the provocation effect.

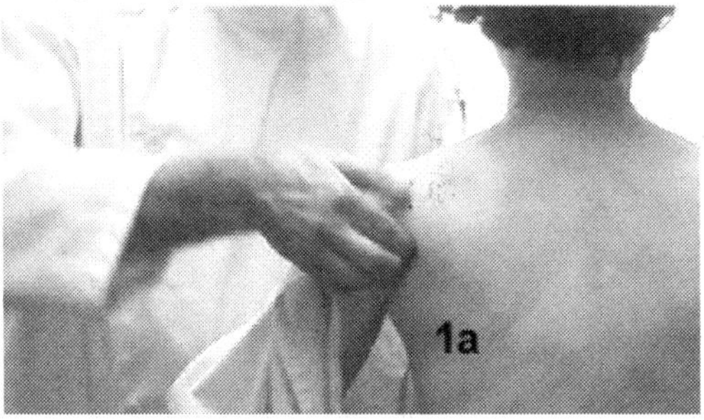

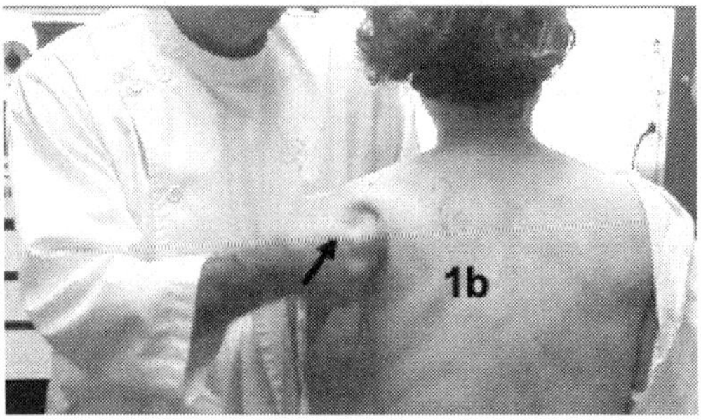

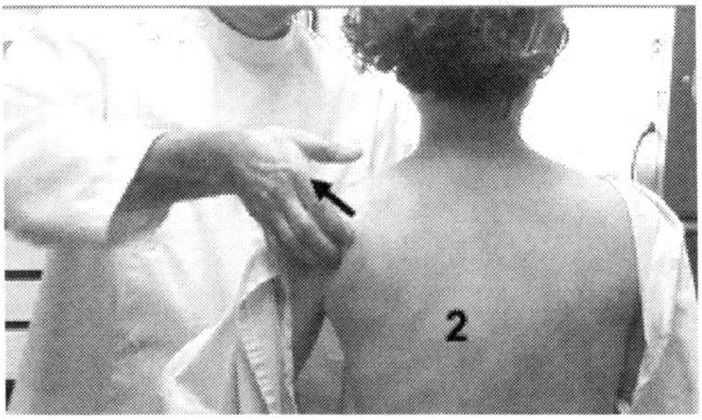

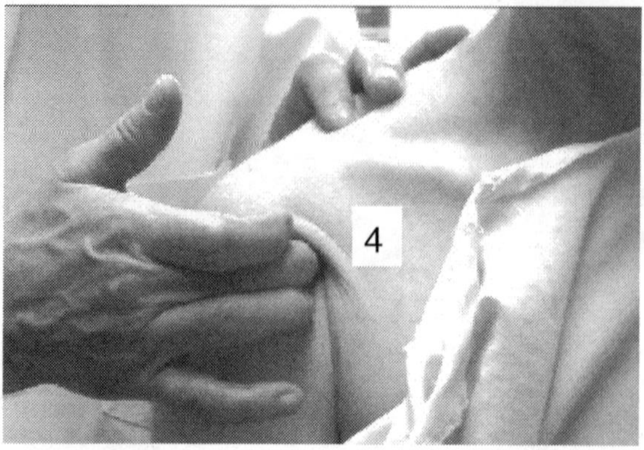

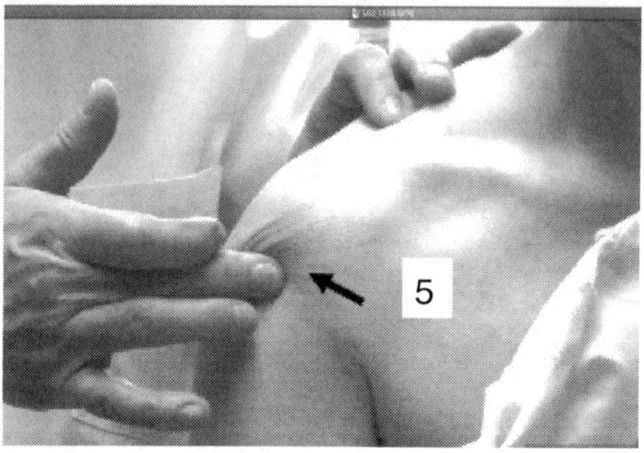

3. Passively abduct the subject's arm and palpate the acromioclavicular joint on the anterior shoulder. Abducting the arm should create a depression there. Place finger there and lower the arm to a natural hanging position.
4. With the finger still in place, drag it anteromedially until you feel the muscle spring back under your stroke.
5. Press and drag the finger (or tool) diagonally across the anterior deltoid toward the acromion until you feel the muscle spring.
6. Pause two minutes.
7. Repeat on opposite side.

Arm Dysfunctions (tennis elbow, golfer's elbow, carpal tunnel syndrome, etc.)

Before treating the arm, one should look for any dysfunction in the neck or shoulder and treat accordingly before commencing the arm protocol. When treating the arm, treat as below on the unaffected or less affected arm first, as usual.

1. Palpate the anterior shoulder, pressing through the anterior deltoid onto the Biceps short head tendon underneath.
2. Drag the tissues beneath your thumb or tool in a medial direction. The motion will naturally stop after rolling over the muscle. Hold the pressure there without releasing the pressure.
3. Reverse direction and roll the tissues laterally and feel the contact roll over the muscle to create the provocation.
4. Flex the arm and palpate the dorsal surface of the forearm. Measure distally from the elbow crease using the index, middle, and ring fingers to locate acupuncture point LI-10, which lies on the Extensor carpi radialis longus. Press deeply on this point until subject feels a strong sensation.
5. Reposition the thumb or tool in an ulnar direction to arrive at the border of the Extensor digitorum and Extensor carpi radialis muscles. If you cannot feel the depression where the two muscles meet, ask the subject to dorsiflex the hand. Press

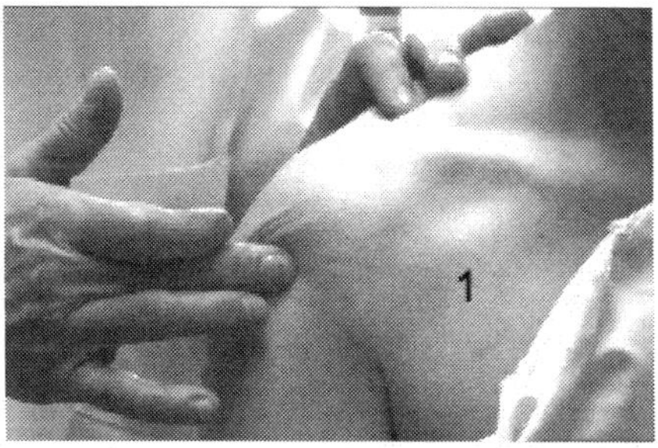

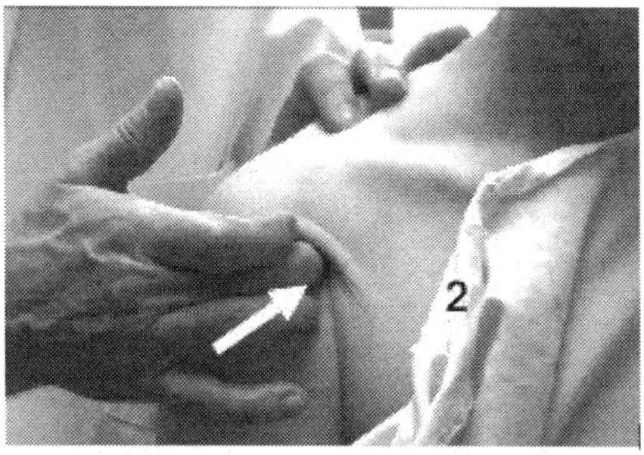

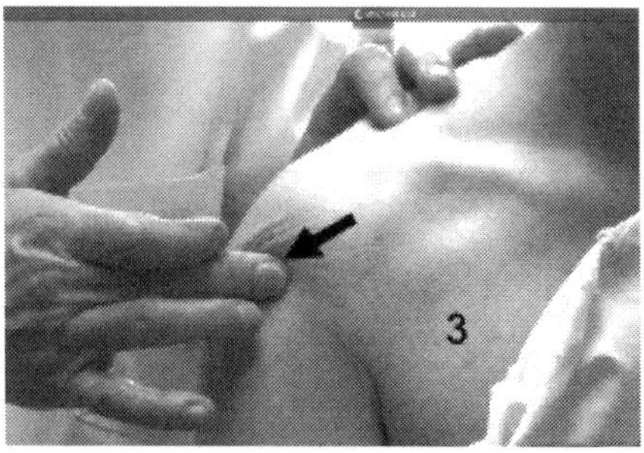

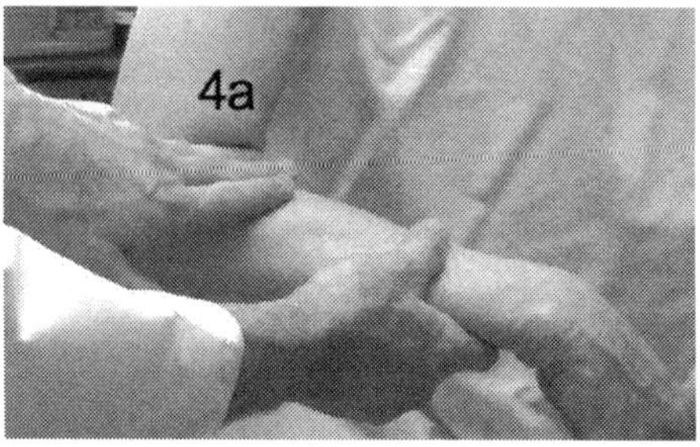

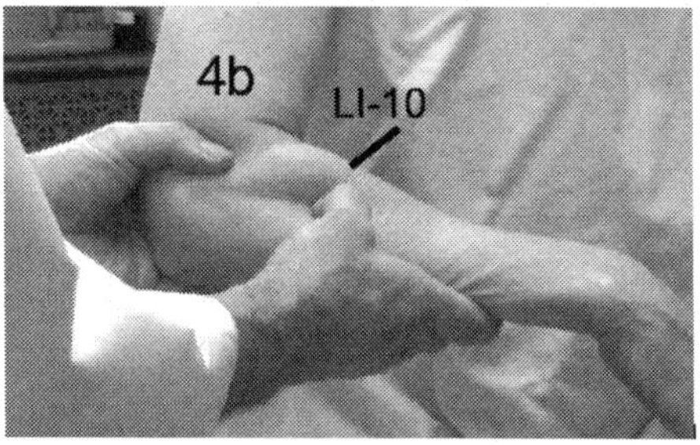

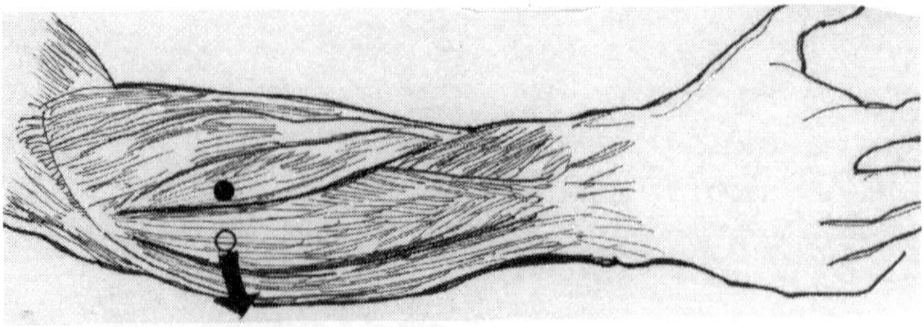

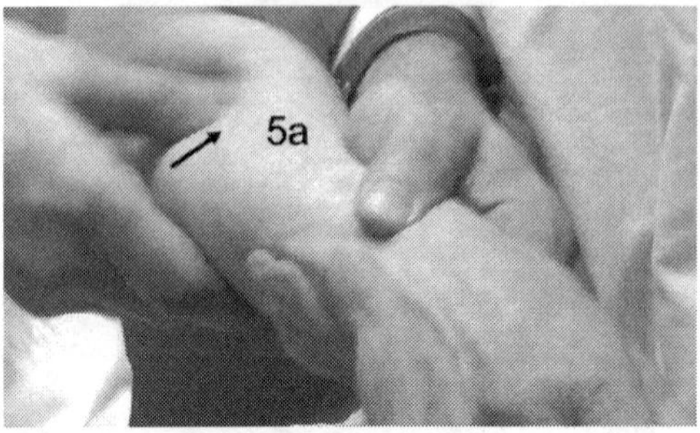

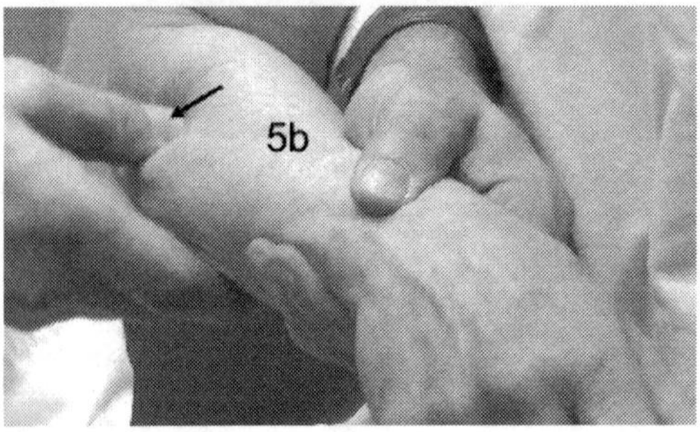

and draw the tissues medially over the Extensor digitorum muscle, press firmly at that spot and reverse direction, rolling toward the ulna over the muscle to end over the Extensor carpi radialis. Provocation at this point will cause the subject's third finger to involuntarily extend.

6. With the subject's arm still flexed, palpate the tendon insertion of the long head of the Triceps on the posterior arm. Draw the tissues medially, press in at the border of the tendon, then release in a lateral direction to create the provocation. This stimulates acupuncture point TW-11.

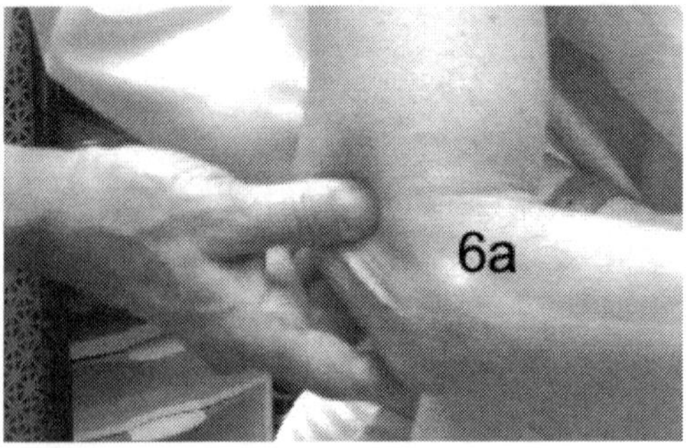

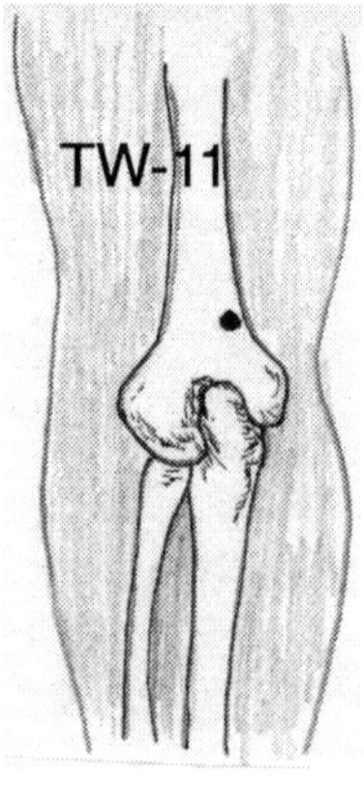

In a muscular subject, it is sometimes necessary to roll back and forth over the tendon several times using the knuckle or a tool, in order to achieve the provocation. Always ask the subject if the characteristic sensation is felt, which is typically somewhere between a short-lived tingle and an ache.

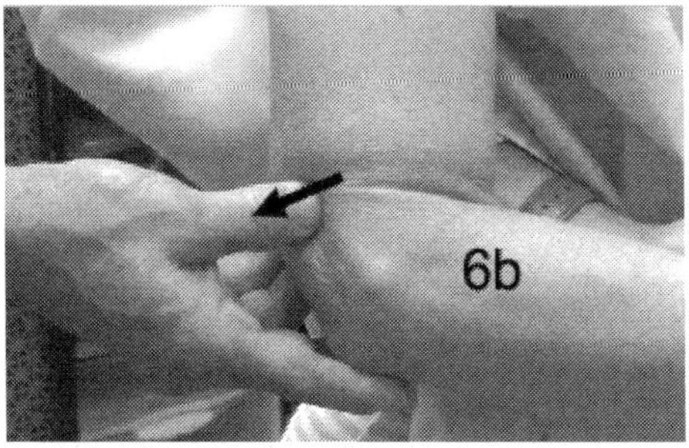

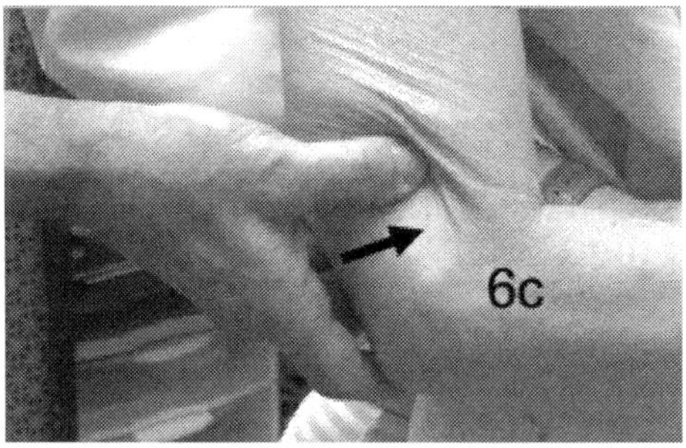

7. Hold subject's hand in a palm-down position. Draw the tissues overlying the Extensor retinaculum toward the ulnar styloid. Then reverse direction and drag toward the radius.

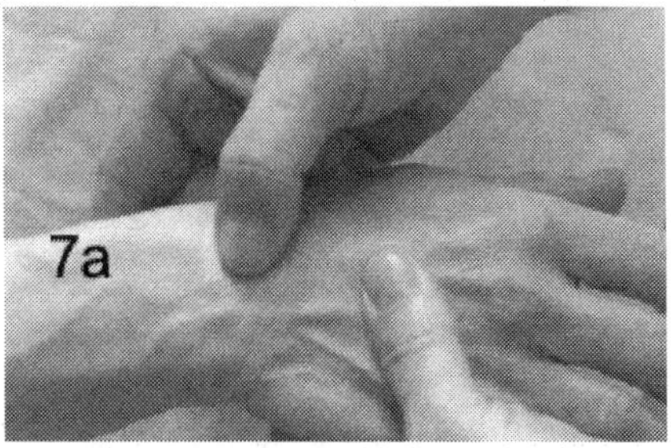

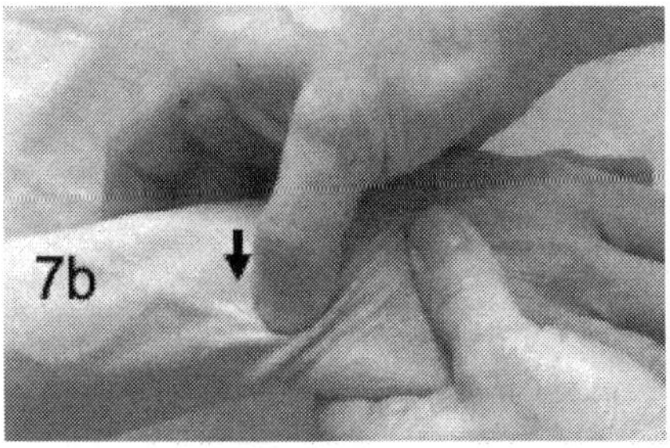

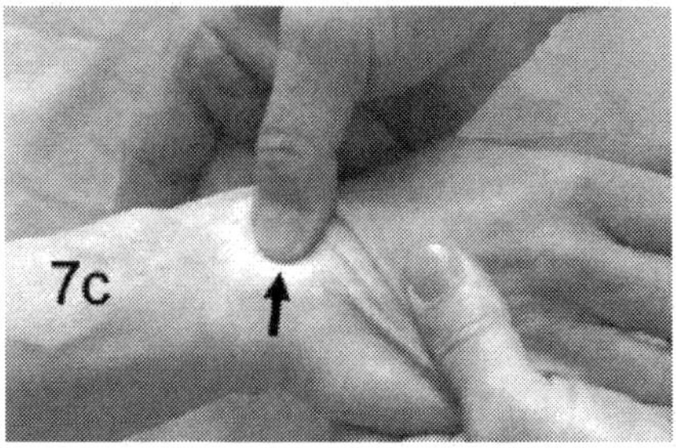

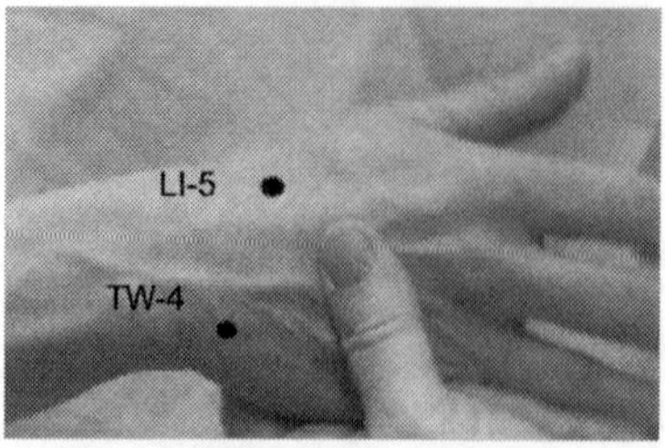

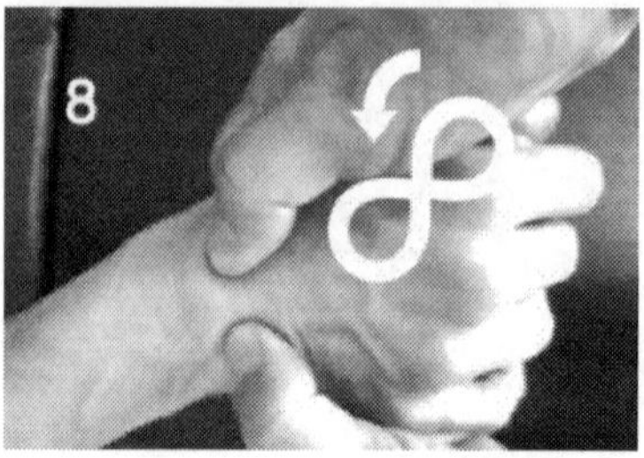

8. Press the thumbs into the depressions where points LI-5 and TW-4 reside. Grip the wrist between the thumbs and the fingers on the palmar side. With subject's wrist slightly flexed and relaxed, passively move the wrist by making a figure-8 motion several times. Finish by giving a gentle tug distally with subject's wrist maintaining flexion, in order to create a momentary traction on the carpal bones.

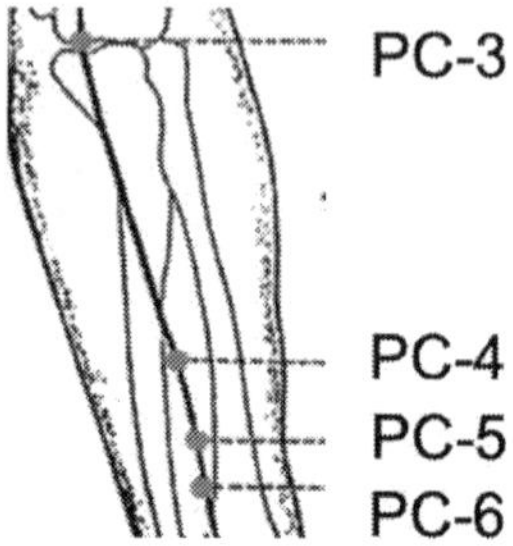

9. Turning subject's hand palm up, palpate the volar surface of the forearm with the thumbs as seen in the illustration. Press on the point PC-4 and draw the thumbs in opposite directions simultaneously, dragging the tissues with them as though parting two panels of curtains. Move distally to press on the point PC-5, then draw the thumbs apart again. Finally, perform the same action over point PC-6, pressing deeply and then drawing in both directions. Subject should feel a strong sensation at deep pressure here.

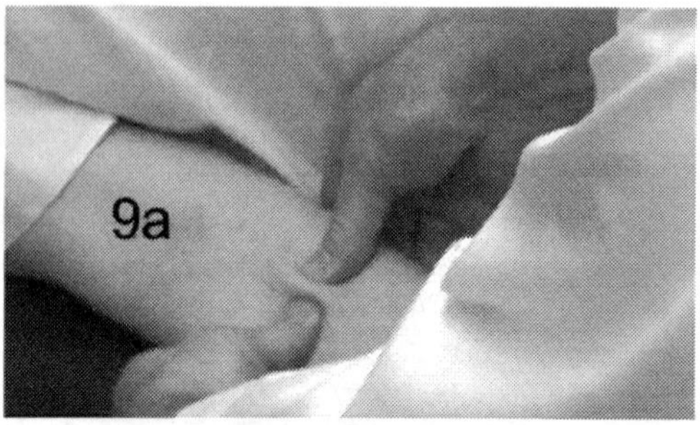

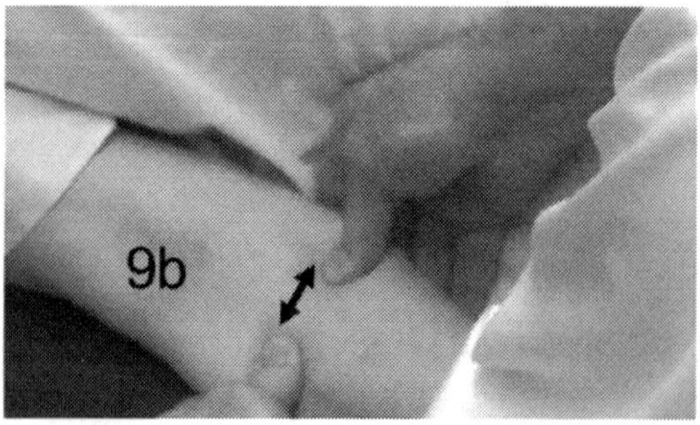

10. Press with the heels of operator's palms against the radial and ulnar surfaces, simultaneously squeezing the tissues back toward the midline, in the opposite order as before, moving proximally in three sets.

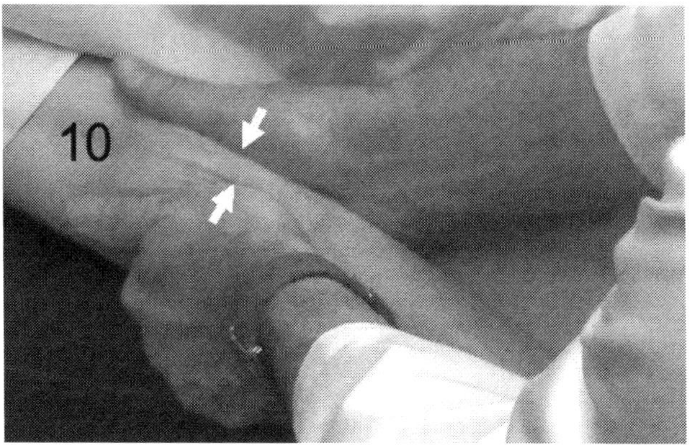

11. Pause two minutes and perform on the other arm.

Knee Dysfunction

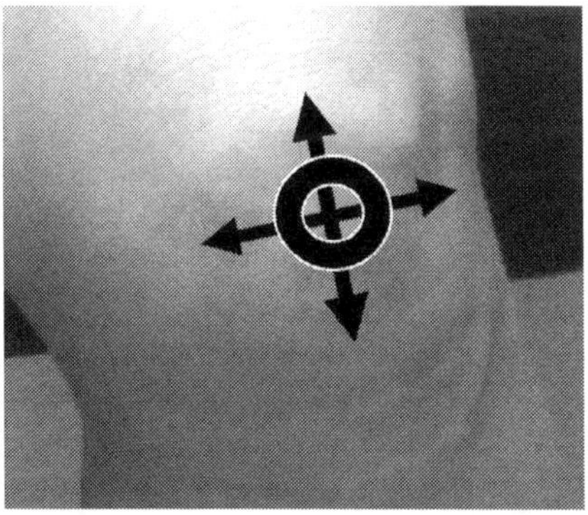

1. Operator stands to side of table facing in a cephalic direction. Treat the unaffected or less affected knee first. Subject in supine position with the leg extended, manipulate the patella several times from side to side and superiorly-inferiorly.

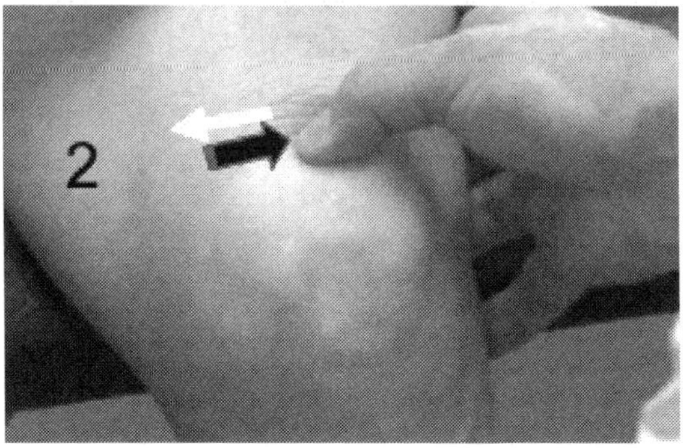

2. Place the thumb over the X-31 point (apex point of the knee), draw tissues laterally and reverse direction, drawing medially until operator feels the patellar tendon make a flipping motion.

3. Slide the thumb diagonally and laterally over the so-called (acupuncture jargon)"eyes of the knee",containing points X-35 and St-35.

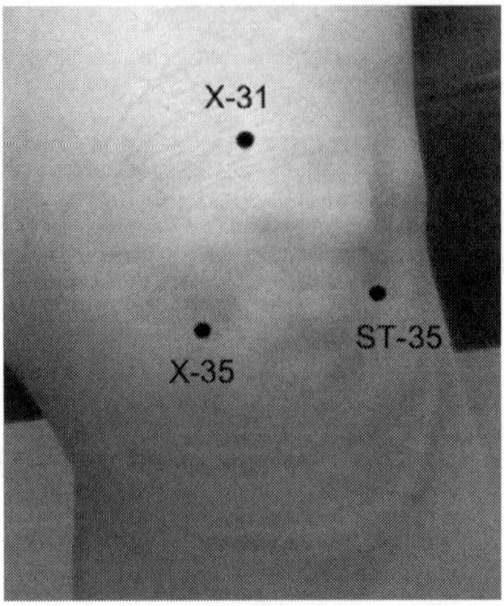

4. Flex the knee and cup the patella with the palm (right hand for left knee, left hand for right knee). Where the thumb contacts the medial surface of the thigh lies point Sp-10. Drag the thumb diagonally in a medial direction across the Vastus medialis, then reverse direction to "spring" the muscle and create the provocation.

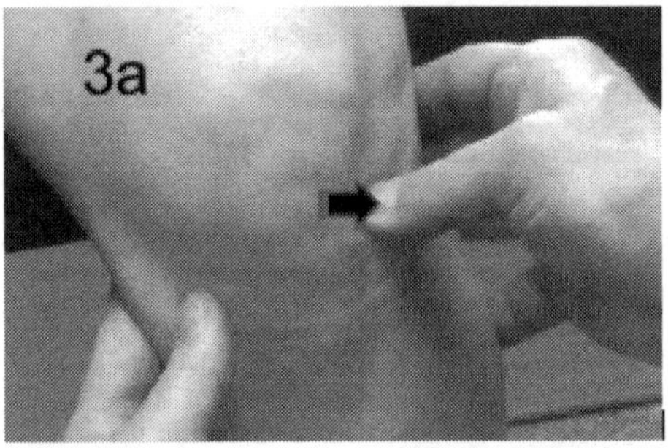

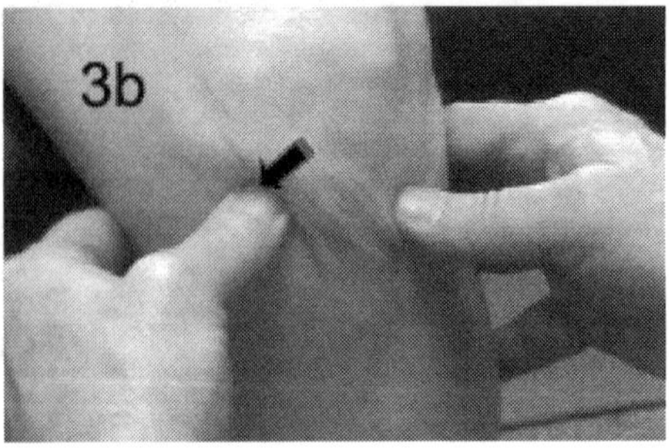

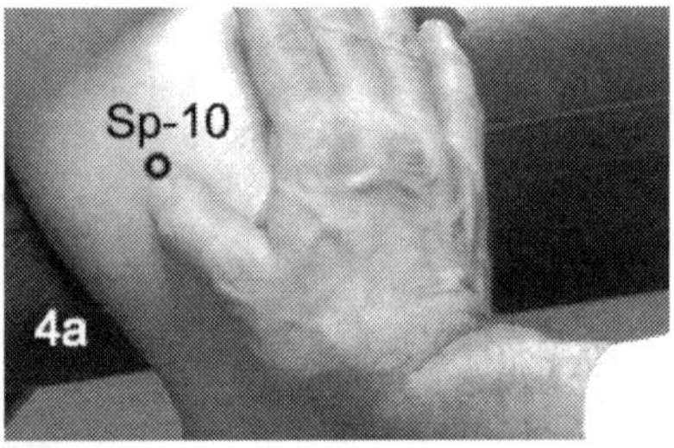

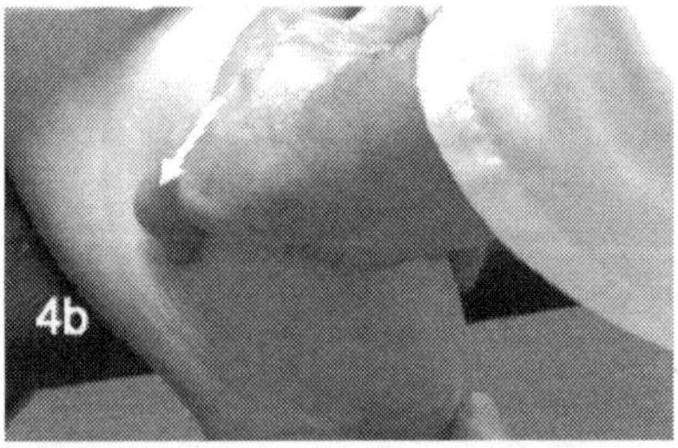

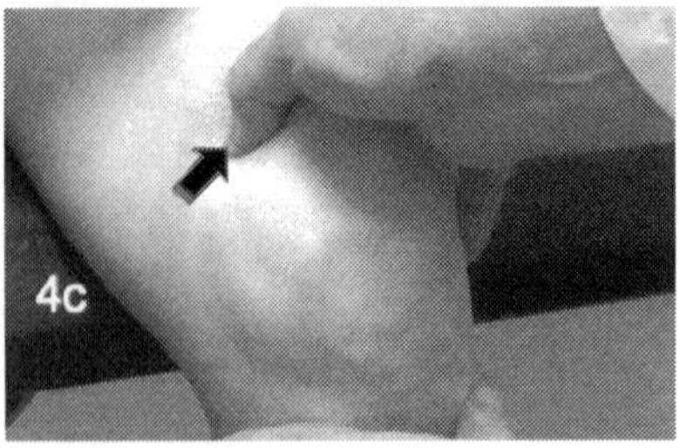

5. Have subject sit with leg dangling over edge of table. With the knee at 90 degrees and relaxed, pull on the ankle to create vertical traction on the knee joint, and passively move the lower leg in small circular motions for a minute. Alternatively, attach an ankle weight to the leg and have the subject perform the movement actively.
6. Subject should rest for 2 minutes before moving or continuing treatment.

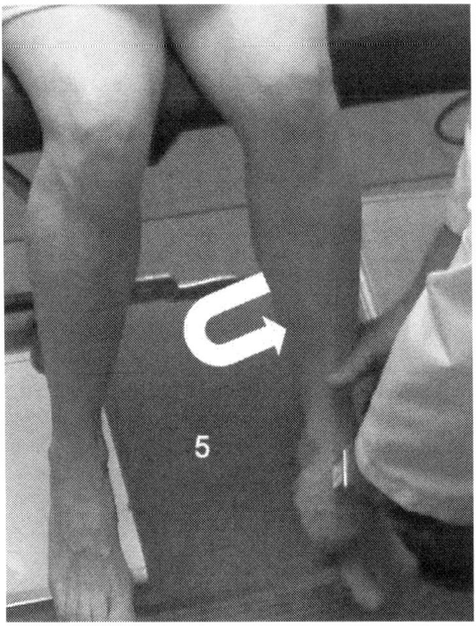

Ankle Dysfunction

As always, treat the unaffected or less affected side first.

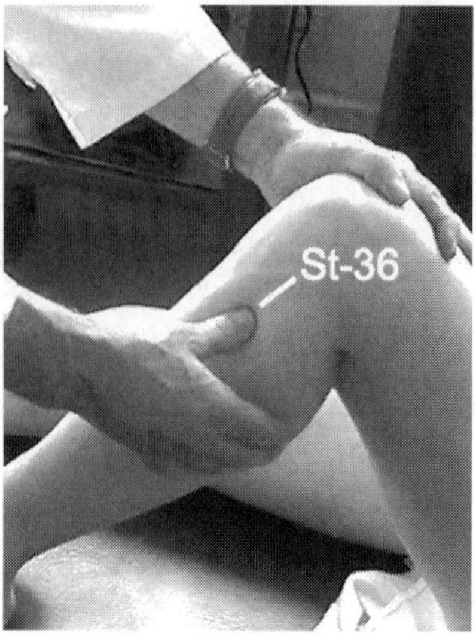

1. With subject supine and the leg flexed at the knee and foot on the table, palpate the anterior Tibialis muscle at a level of four fingers' width distal to the lower border of the patella, on the lateral side of the tibia. The point St-36 is located here. Have subject relax the leg and press over the St-36 point and roll laterally across the muscle. Then reverse direction and roll medially until the thumb or tool contacts the tibia[93]. Perform this 3-4 times to ensure that the provocation has been made.

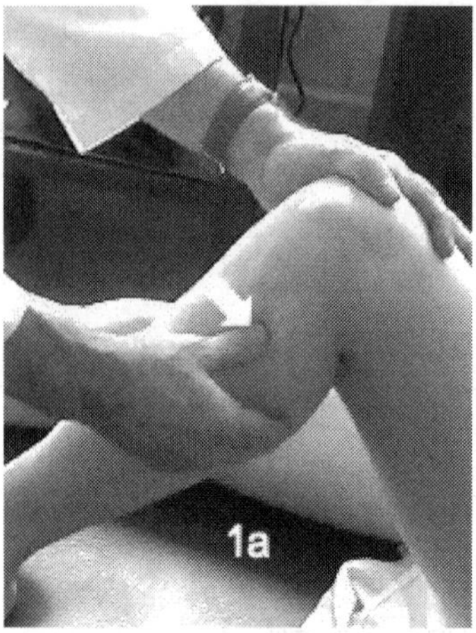

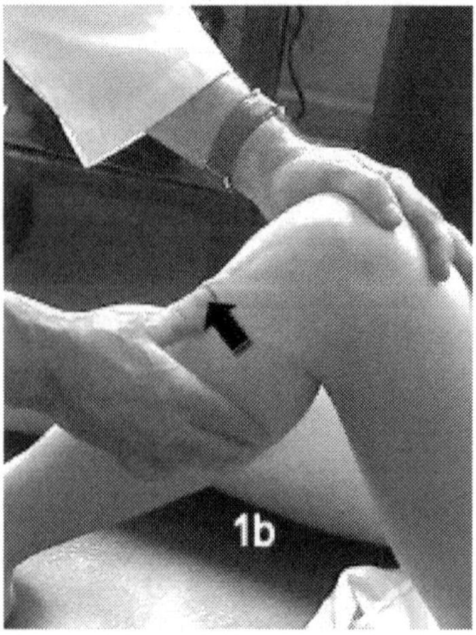

2. Have subject extend the leg and rest it on the table. Palpate the lateral Malleolus. Keeping a firm pressure, draw the tissues distally,

[93] If the muscle tone is very firm, a knuckle can be used instead of the thumb.

then reverse direction, pulling them in a plantar direction and then posteriorly, creating a circling of the Malleolus. Subject should be able to feel the provocation.

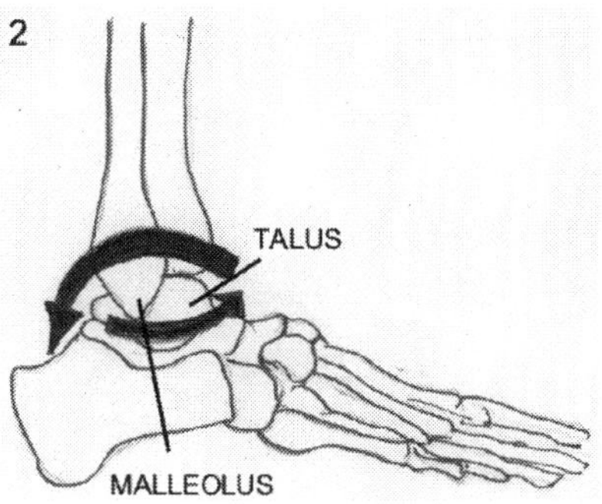

3. Press the thumb into the depression at the tarsal sinus on the medial side of the Talus. Press the index finger into the symmetrical depression on the lateral side. The hand will be gripping each side of the Talus[94]. Grip firmly while using the other hand to grip the ball of the foot to dorsiflex the toes. Maintaining a firm grip on the ball of the foot, further dorsiflex the foot and rotate it in each direction, making a circle while maintaining pressure at the Talus. Holding the foot in maximum dorsiflexion, raise the elbow of the arm gripping the foot and perform a short thrusting motion against the contact points while pushing

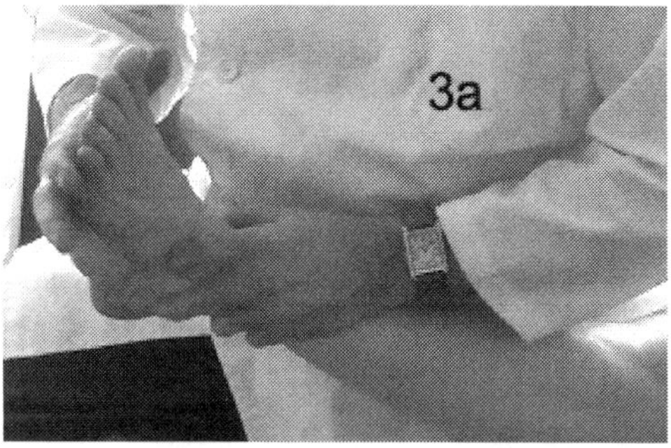

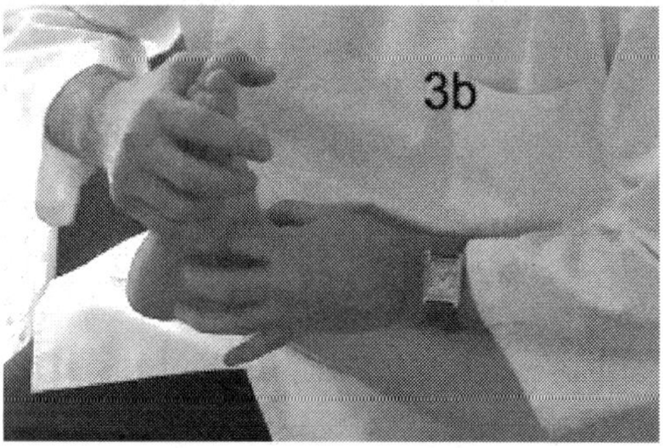

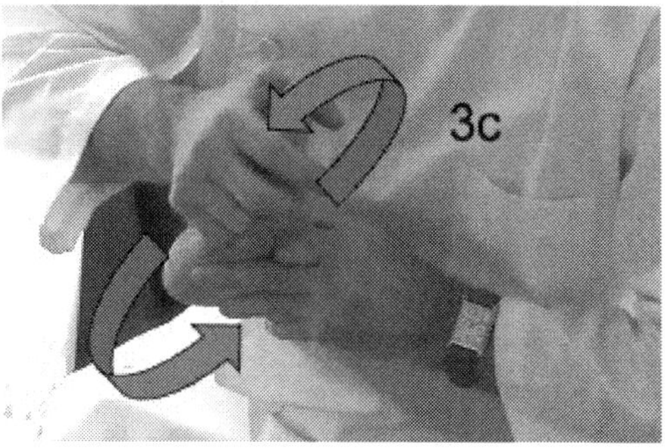

[94] Simultaneously stimulating points LV-4 and GB-40, affecting the Deep Peroneal nerve and the Intermediate dorsal cutaneous nerve, respectively.

the ball of the foot toward the ankle. Dropping the elbow allows a more efficient use of leverage, directing the force of the long bones of the arm against the subject's ankle joint.

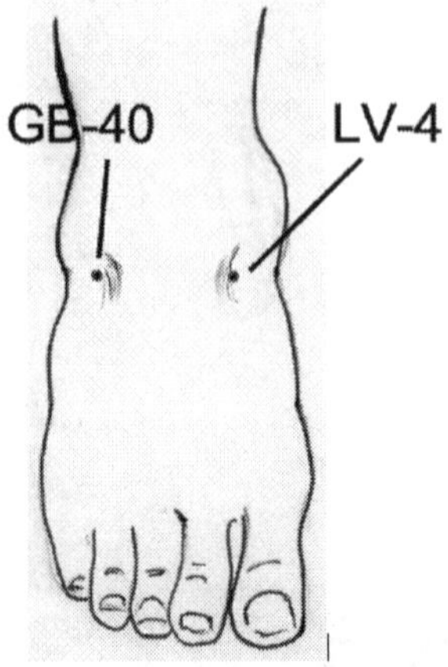

4.Lower the foot to the table, and cup one hand under the calcaneus and grip the distal part of the foot with the other hand. Keeping the foot close to the table, pull the foot in extension and slight plantar flexion. While maintaining traction on the ankle, give a tug on the calcaneus to momentarily gap the tarsal bones and stretch the fascia.

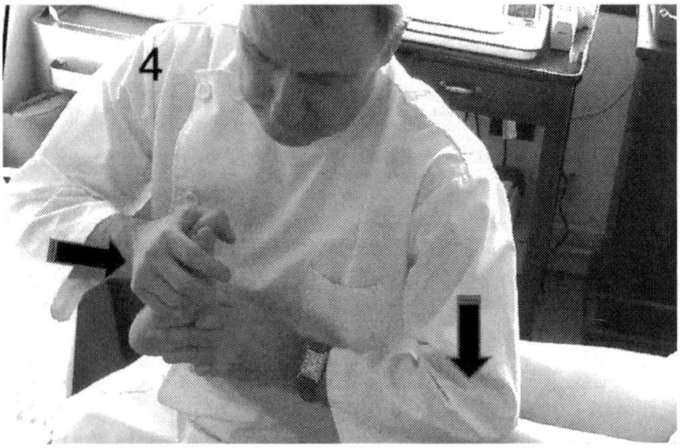

5. Allow the leg to rest for two minutes before proceeding further.

Allergies / Sinusitis Protocol

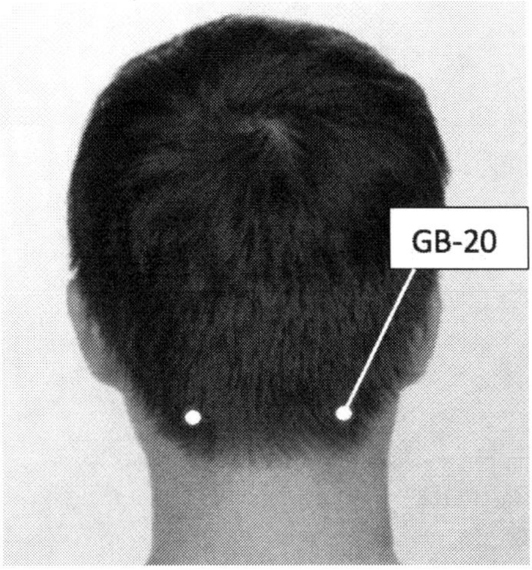

Best results are achieved by performing the neck protocol first.

1. Subject in the supine position, locate point GB-20 midway between the mastoid bone and the suboccipital depression below the protuberance (see illustration). Stimulate with pressure, electrical stimulation, or other tool. Point will typically be tender to palpation with this condition. Provocation is complete when subject vocalizes pain or a strong sensation. Turn subject's head to the opposite side as you treat the point. Treat both sides.

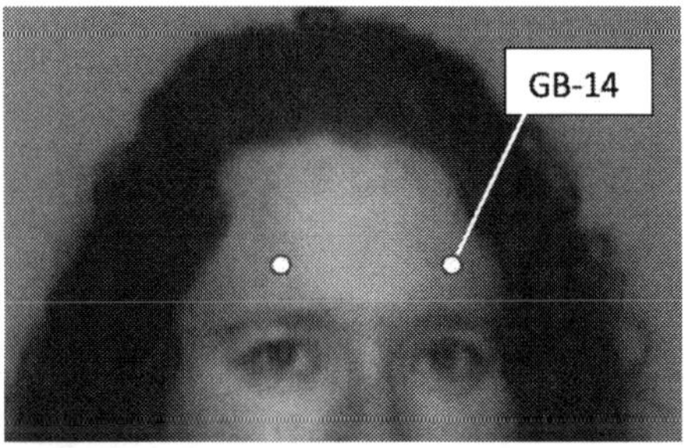

2. Locate point GB-14, approximately one thumb width superior to the midpoint of the eyebrow. Stimulate this point in a circular motion if using a finger.

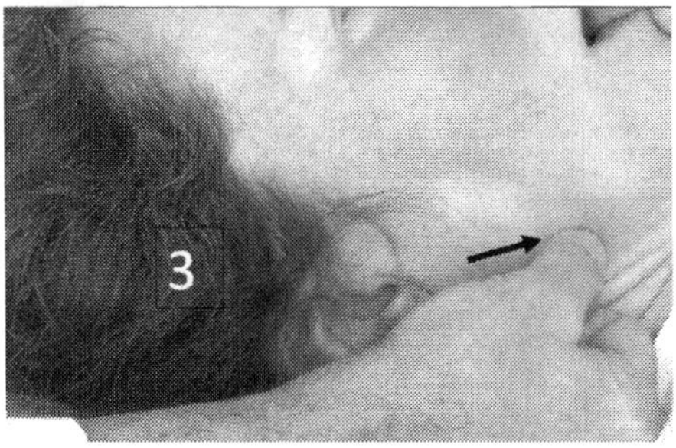

3. Place finger or tool on point St-6, anterior and superior to the angle of the jaw on the prominence of the Masseter muscle (can locate by having subject clench teeth). Draw the tissues posteriorly towards the mandibular angle and then reverse direction to arrive at point St-5, as in the illustration.
4. Repeat on opposite side.

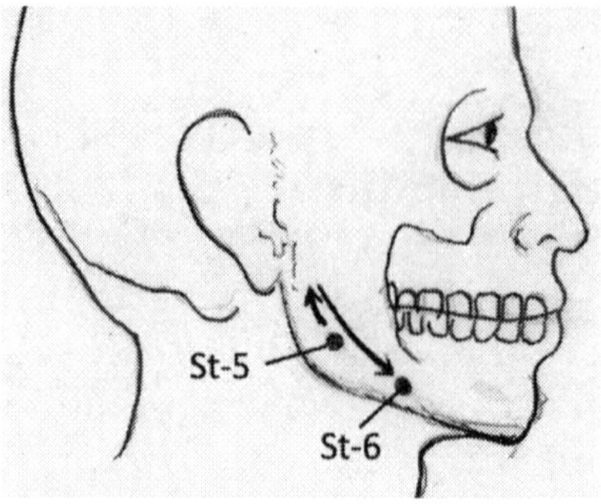

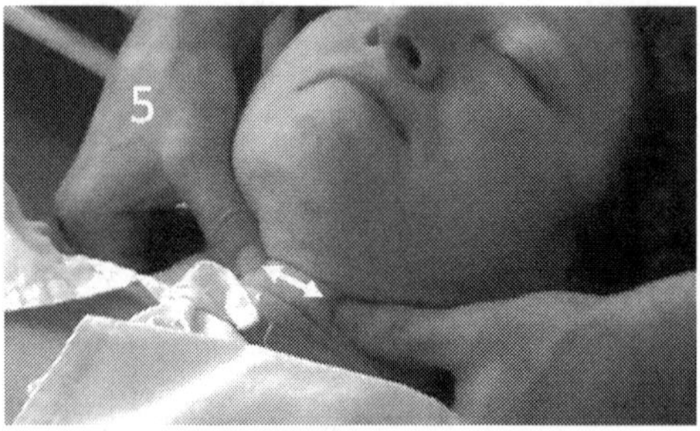

5.Making gentle movements, move the cricoid cartilage left and right several times. If it is rigid, wait a few minutes and try again. If it is not free by the third try, abandon this step until the next treatment.

(Continued on next page)

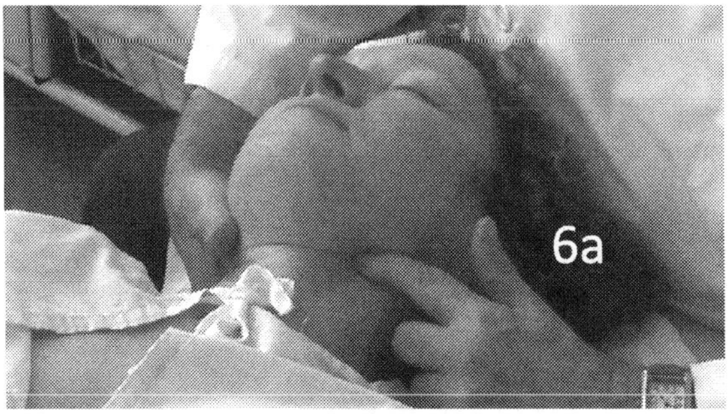

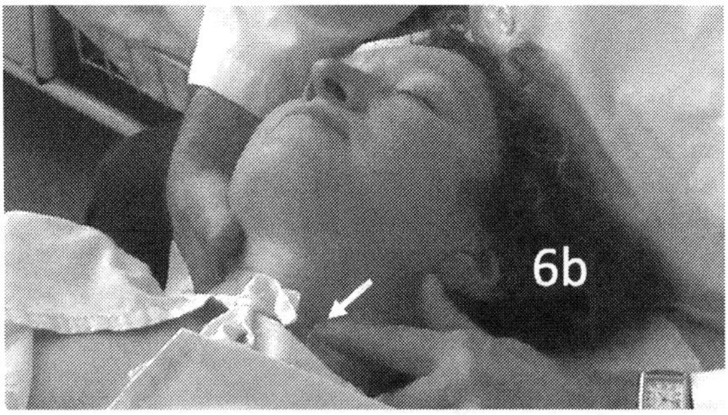

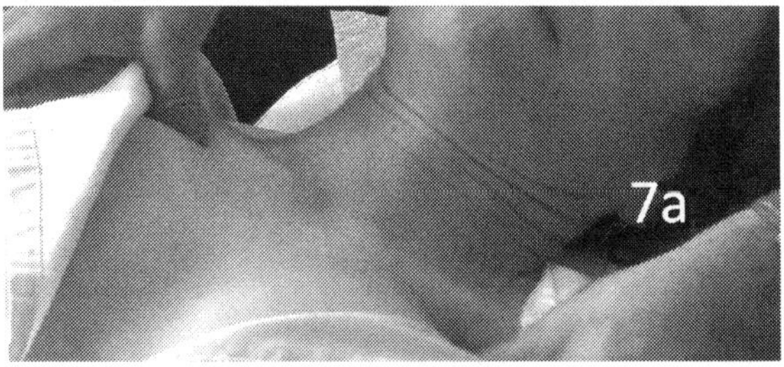

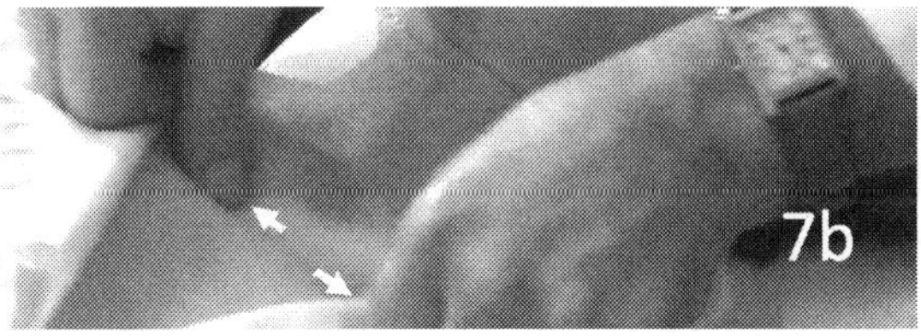

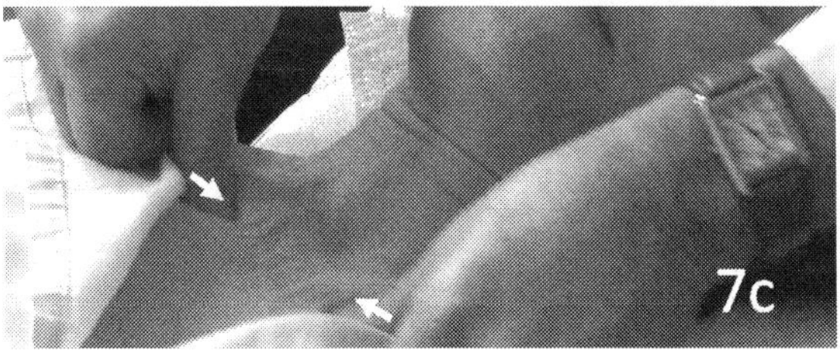

6. Move the tissues on both sides of the cricoid cartilage in a caudal direction, in one stroking motion down each side. This stimulates points St-9 and St-10. **Deep pressure is not used**, but a short, quick stroke that stretches the tissues.

7. Press into the first intercostal space at the most lateral positions and rub all along the superior aspect of the second rib[95], working your way medially. When you reach the most medial position, press the sternoclavicular joint[96] with both thumbs and draw the tissues laterally along the clavicle (Fig. 7b), then reverse direction and stroke in a medial direction (Fig. 7c). Work quickly, as this point will be tender.

---

[95] Chapman's reflexes for the sinuses.

[96] Chapman's nasal reflexes.

8. With subject's head turned to his right, lightly squeeze the Sternocleidomastoid muscle at the angle of the mandible. Reposition the fingers inferiorly and repeat. Continue until the entire lymphatic chain in this region has been stimulated. When operator reaches the clavicle, the procedure is repeated on the right side, with subject's head turned left.

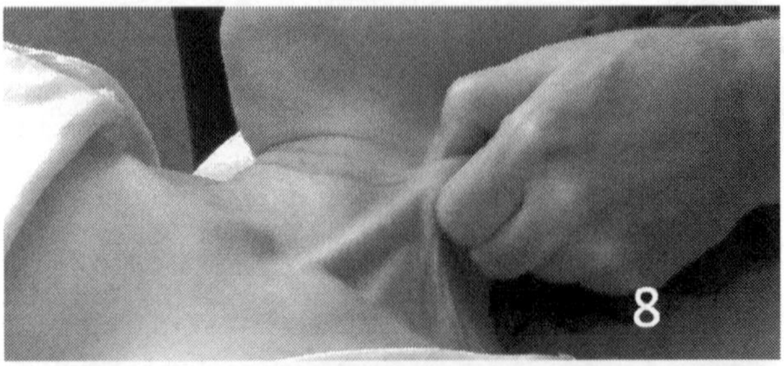

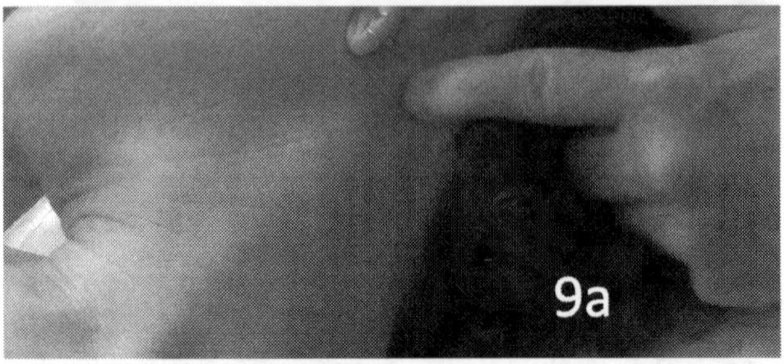

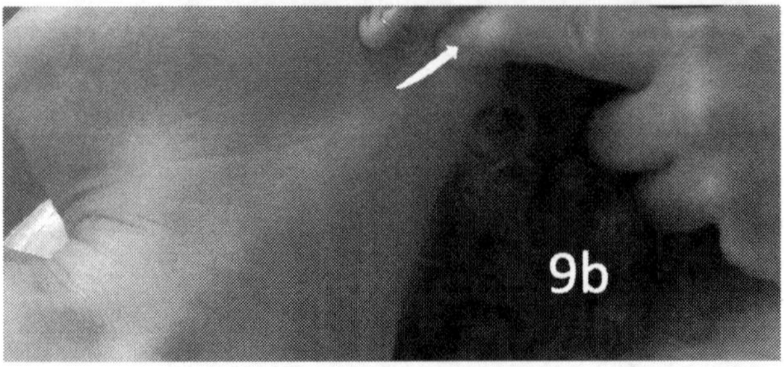

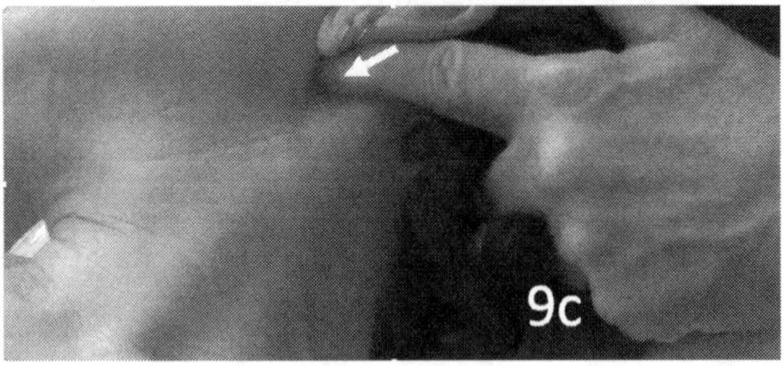

9. Place the index finger (or tool, if it is padded) on the left mastoid bone (9a) and draw the tissues in a cephalic direction (9b), then reverse direction so that the finger slips into the depression behind the earlobe between the mastoid process and the angle of the mandible, which houses point TW-17 (9c).
10. Repeat the same movement on the right side, and allow subject to rest for two minutes.

Lower Respiratory dysfunction / Asthma

Subject lies prone. Operator stands at end of table facing caudal direction.

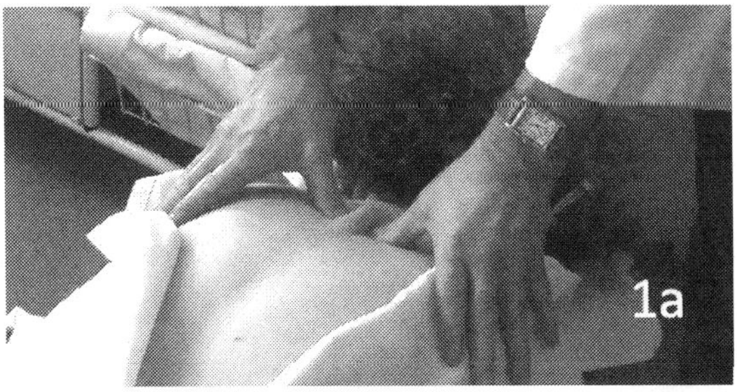

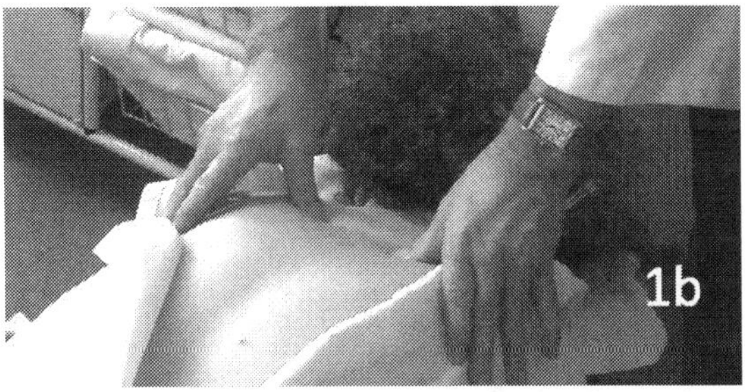

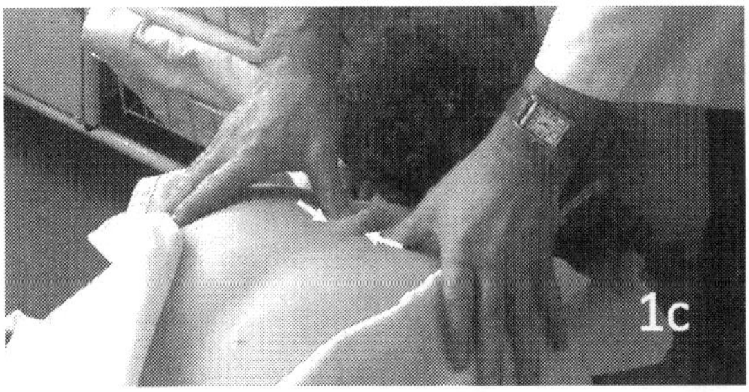

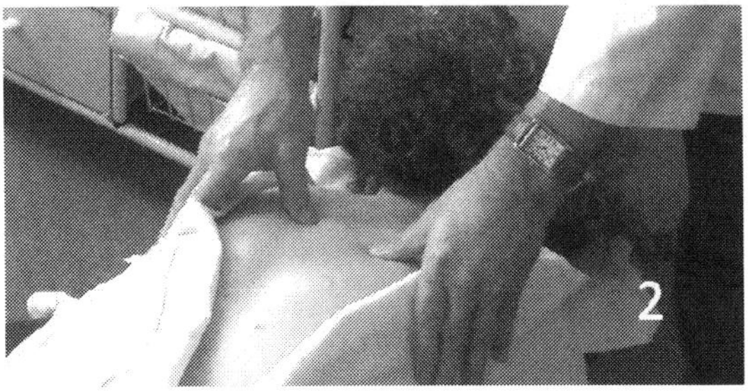

1. Begin with the thumbs each over the T2-T3 junction with the tips of the thumbs almost touching under the T2 spinous process. Pressing down, the thumbs are drawn apart laterally to stretch the skin and fascia and roll it over the prominence of the Longissimus muscle, which can be felt beneath the more superficial Trapezius. This stimulates both the vertebral points and associated point of the lungs (UB-12) at that spinal level. Draw the thumbs apart as far as a hand width lateral to the midline, then reverse direction, drawing the tissues toward the midline.
2. Move caudally to the T3-T4 junction and repeat the same maneuver at that level. This stimulates the vertebral points and the other associated bladder point (UB-13) for the lungs.

3. Have subject roll over to supine position. Locate the space between the sternocostal junctions of the third and fourth ribs. Press in with a finger or tool and draw the tissues medially over the border of the sternum. Then drag the tissues laterally to create the provocation[97]. Treat both left and right. This will likely be tender in any respiratory condition.

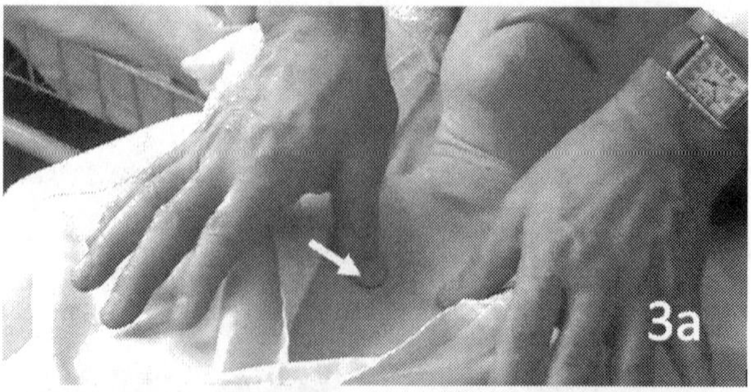

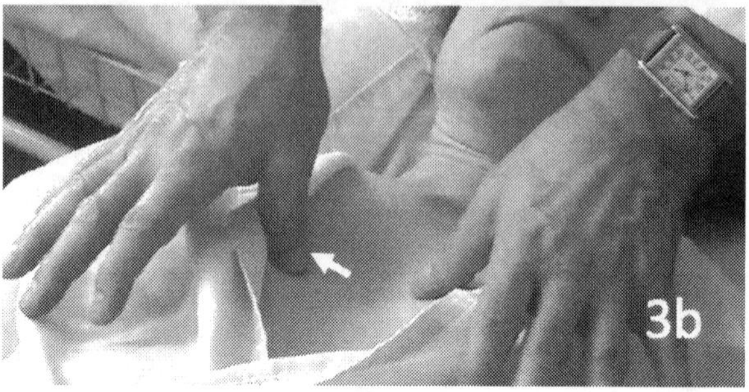

4. Change position inferiorly to the space between the fourth and fifth ribs and repeat the maneuver.
5. Place finger or tool against the inferior border of the bottom rib on the left side at approximately the midway point between the sternum and the free rib. Have subject inhale and

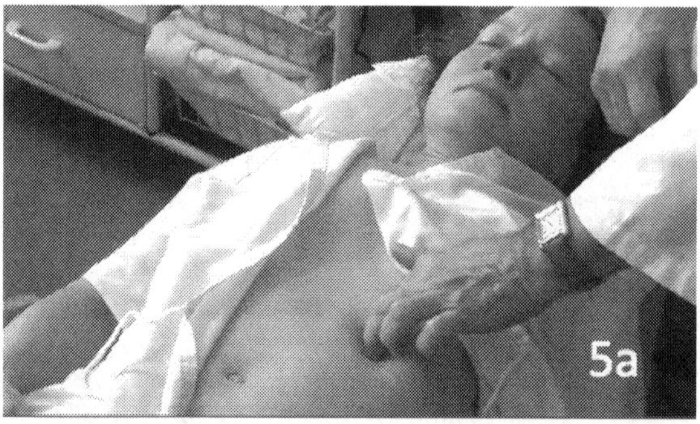

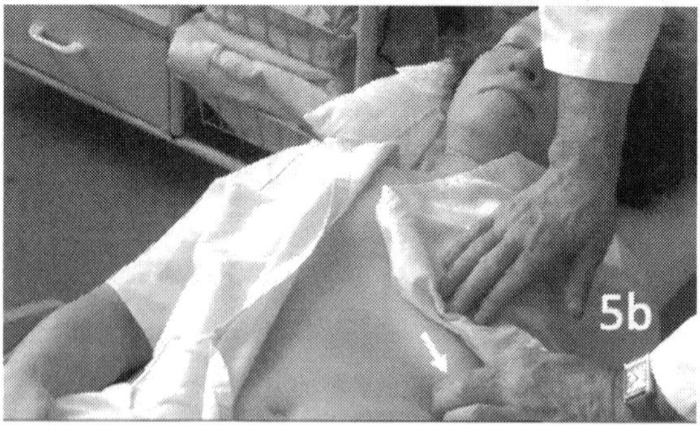

[97] The provocation could be made with the opposite sequence, dragging the tissues laterally and then medially over the sternal border. Both methods seem to be effective.

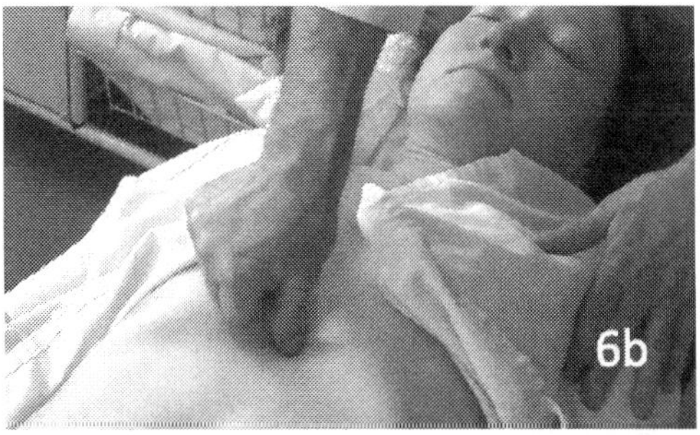

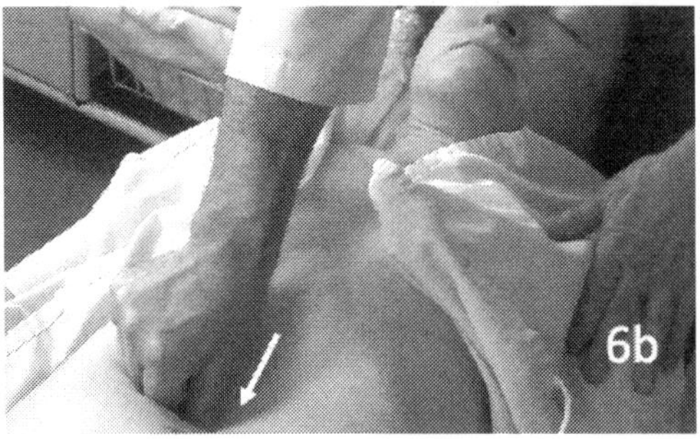

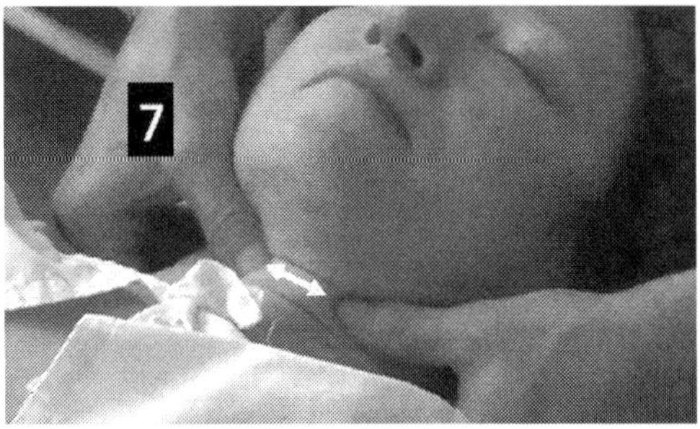

exhale. When the exhalation is complete, curl under the rib and stroke along the rib obliquely across the insertion of the Rectus abdominis. Repeat on the right side.

6. Place finger or tool about one inch inferior to the xiphoid process. Without any deep pressure, draw the tissues inferiorly in the direction of the umbilicus.

7. Finish with trachea provocation: Making gentle movements, move the cricoid cartilage left and right several times. Then, while maintaining a grip on it, move it in a caudal direction a very short distance, using no force.

8. Have subject rest for two minutes with no further stimulation before moving.

The following is a handout given to patients when receiving Uni-Syn treatment.

A Few Words About Your Treatment…

You will have a number of points treated with gentle rolling movements that stimulate clusters of nerve reflexes and acupuncture points. This allows information carried on the nerves to be routed to the areas they need to go. This will be done in a sequence with pauses between the point stimulation. This allows the brain to understand the signal created in the muscle and to send a signal of its own back to the tissues.

You may experience sensations of heat, chilling, or shaking as a result of the treatment. Some of your symptoms may become temporarily worse. Such effects are not harmful and are a sign that the body is responding.

To get the best results from your treatment:

- **Drink plenty of water** on the day of treatment and after.
- **Walk** for 10-20 minutes, but **avoid strenuous exercise** for a day or two.
- **Every 30 minutes, get up and move around** on the day of treatment. Allow a maximum of a half hour for sitting without getting up for a minute. If driving, stop every half hour and walk around the car.
- **Keep your limbs uncrossed.** The healing signal can be interrupted this way, believe it or not.
- **Take warm, not hot, baths or showers** on the day of treatment. Avoid hot or cold packs also.
- **No additional treatment for 7 days after** (acupuncture, chiropractic, massage, etc.). Your session here has reset your body's fields allowing it to heal itself. Interfering with that new message hampers progress.
- **The body is on a 7-day healing cycle** and needs this time to respond. Another session will probably be scheduled in a week to build on the previous treatment.

18

SUMMARY of UNI-SYN

TEN RULES FOR GOOD RESULTS

1. **Observe the dual polarity of anabolic and catabolic effects.** First differentiate between excess and deficient conditions and stimulate accordingly, as per #2.
2. **Strong stimulation for acute cases, weak stimulation for chronic.**
   - Acupuncture: Sedation for acute; tonification for chronic
   - Hydrotherapy: Long cold or hot application to sedate; short to tonify
   - Manual: Strong technic/joint mobilization for acute; soft tissue technic for chronic
   - Electrotherapy: Strong stimulation for acute (higher amperage for transdermal; thermal setting for short wave; more impulses of piezoelectricity[98]; etc.). Weaker stimulation for chronic (mild currents, non-thermal settings, fewer impulses)
   - Botanical medicines: Pharmacological doses for acute; small doses for chronic
   - Homeopathic medicines: High potencies for acute; medium to low potencies for chronic (very low in protracted doses if tissue changes are present)
   - Chromotherapy: Opposing-action colors for acute (blue for inflammation, etc.); same-action colors for chronic (red, etc.)

98 Curiously, tonification and sedation with piezoelectric stimulation does not seem to be as critical, because the body tends to create the needed reaction—stimulating or inhibiting—as the brain decides. Whether this is due to piezoelectricity speaking the body's "language" or not remains to be established.

3. **Provocation of the points must create a piezoelectric effect in the tissues,** whether stimulation is by hand, needle, or electricity (or piezoelectricity itself).
4. **Treat often for acute; less often for chronic.**
5. **Observe periodicity and its effects.**
    - Make provocations up to seven times at a site and pause. If pain remains after 2-3 minutes, repeat. Make a third set of provocations after another pause if needed.
    - Allow rest of 2-3 minutes between provocation of each region of the body, and after end of treatment
    - Any continuous treatment (electrotherapy, etc.) to be applied for 21 minutes.
    - Treatment at seven-day intervals for chronic conditions, with no other therapy in between (e.g.: chiropractic in addition to acupuncture, or acupuncture in addition to massage, etc.).
    - Observe that different phases of healing occur at 7, 14, and 21 days; also at seven weeks, seven months, and seven years.
5. **Give as little treatment as possible.**
6. **Always treat spinal points in addition to distal or local areas.**
7. **Always treat bilaterally and treat the asymptomatic or unaffected side of the body before treating the affected side.** Same applies to the less painful side if the problem is bilateral. Provocation of the opposite side engages the brain to accept the treatment of the affected or worse area.
8. **Treat anteriorly as well as posteriorly.** Treat anterior points that correspond to the pertinent points on the posterior. Provocation on both front and back of the thorax excites the spinal cord, and by that means enlists the myotomes, dermatomes, sclerotomes, etc.—multiple levels of provocation are possible.
9. **Monitor for changes.** If tender points lose their tenderness during the treatment, **end that session for the day.** According to the laws of Polarity and Periodicity, continued provocation would cause the pain to return (If giving oral medicine, **discontinue if symptoms become suddenly and dramatically better or worse.** The

healing response has been engaged, and further provocation / dosing will keep trying to re-start that process and will delay resolution).

10. **Act as a conduit** for whatever greater force you can imagine and do not feel as though the healing comes from you.

Made in the USA
Monee, IL
05 November 2026

67812850R00125